A Manager's Guide to the Design and Conduct of Clinical Trials

A MANAGER'S GUIDE TO THE DESIGN AND CONDUCT OF CLINICAL TRIALS

Second Edition

Phillip I. Good, Ph.D.

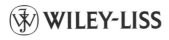

A JOHN WILEY & SONS, INC., PUBLICATION

Copyright © 2006 by John Wiley & Sons, Inc. All rights reserved.

Published by John Wiley & Sons, Inc., Hoboken, New Jersey.
Published simultaneously in Canada.

No part of this publication may be reproduced, stored in a retrieval system, or transmitted in any form or by any means, electronic, mechanical, photocopying, recording, scanning, or otherwise, except as permitted under Section 107 or 108 of the 1976 United States Copyright Act, without either the prior written permission of the Publisher, or authorization through payment of the appropriate per-copy fee to the Copyright Clearance Center, Inc., 222 Rosewood Drive, Danvers, MA 01923, (978) 750-8400, fax (978) 750-4470, or on the web at www.copyright.com. Requests to the Publisher for permission should be addressed to the Permissions Department, John Wiley & Sons, Inc., 111 River Street, Hoboken, NJ 07030, (201) 748-6011, fax (201) 748-6008, or online at http://www.wiley.com/go/permission.

Limit of Liability/Disclaimer of Warranty: While the publisher and author have used their best efforts in preparing this book, they make no representations or warranties with respect to the accuracy or completeness of the contents of this book and specifically disclaim any implied warranties of merchantability or fitness for a particular purpose. No warranty may be created or extended by sales representatives or written sales materials. The advice and strategies contained herein may not be suitable for your situation. You should consult with a professional where appropriate. Neither the publisher nor author shall be liable for any loss of profit or any other commercial damages, including but not limited to special, incidental, consequential, or other damages.

For general information on our other products and services or for technical support, please contact our Customer Care Department within the United States at (800) 762-2974, outside the United States at (317) 572-3993 or fax (317) 572-4002.

Wiley also publishes its books in a variety of electronic formats. Some content that appears in print may not be available in electronic formats. For more information about Wiley products, visit our web site at www.wiley.com.

Library of Congress Cataloging-in-Publication Data:

Good, Phillip I.
    A manager's guide to the design and conduct of clinical trials / Phillip Good.–2nd ed.
      p. cm.
    Includes bibliographical references and index.
    ISBN-13: 978-0-471-78870-6 (cloth)
    ISBN-10: 0-471-78870-8 (cloth)
    1. Clinical trials. I. Title
   R853.C55G65 2006
   610.72′4—dc22

2005056950

Printed in the United States of America.

10 9 8 7 6 5 4 3 2

This book has benefited from a number of reviewers. Those I'm at liberty to name are Bernarr Pardo for his excellent advice on data management and David Salsburg.

Contents

1 Cut Costs and Increase Profits **1**
    No Excuse for the Wastage **1**
    Front-Loaded Solution **2**
    Downsizing **3**
    Think Transnational **3**
    A Final Word **4**

2 Guidelines **7**
    Start with Your Reports **7**
    The Wrong Way **9**
    Keep It in the Computer **9**
    Don't Push the River **10**
    KISS **11**
    Plug the Holes as They Arise **12**
    Pay for Results, Not Intentions **13**
    Plan, Do, Then Check **13**

PART I PLAN 15

3 Prescription for Success **17**
    Plan **17**
        A. Predesign Phase **17**
        B. Design the Trials **17**
    Do **19**
        C. Obtain Regulatory Agency Approval for the Trials **19**
        D. Form the Implementation Team **19**

  E. Line Up Your Panel of Physicians **19**
  F. Develop the Data Entry Software **19**
  G. Test the Software **20**
  H. Train **20**
  I. Recruit Patients **20**
  J. Set Up External Review Committees **20**
  K. Conduct the Trials **20**
  L. Develop Suite of Programs for Use in Data Analysis **20**
  M. Analyze and Interpret the Data **21**
 Check **21**
  N. Complete the Submission **21**

4 Staffing for Success **23**
 The People You Need **23**
  Design Team **23**
  Obtain Regulatory Approval for the Trials **25**
  Track Progress **25**
  Implementation Team **26**
  Develop Data Entry Software **26**
  Test the Software **27**
  Line Up Your Panel of Physicians **28**
  External Laboratories **28**
  Site Coordinators **28**
  External Review Committees **29**
  Recruit and Enroll Patients **29**
  Transnational Trials **30**
  Conduct the Trials **30**
  Programs for Data Analysis **30**
  Analyze and Interpret the Data **31**
 The People You Don't Need **31**
 For Further Information **33**

5 Design Decisions **35**
 Should the Study Be Performed? **36**
 Should the Trials Be Transnational? **37**
 Study Objectives **37**
 End Points **38**
  Secondary End Points **39**
  Should We Proceed with a Full-Scale Trial? **41**
  Tertiary End Points **41**
  Baseline Data **41**

Who Will Collect the Data? **41**
Quality Control **42**
Study Population **44**
Timing **45**
Closure **46**
  Planned Closure **46**
  Unplanned Closure **46**
Be Defensive. Review, Rewrite, Review Again **49**
Checklist for Design **50**
Budgets and Expenditures **50**
For Further Information **51**

6 Trial Design **55**
Baseline Measurements **56**
Controlled Randomized Clinical Trials **57**
  Randomized Trials **58**
  Blocked Randomization **59**
  Stratified Randomization **60**
  Single- vs. Double-Blind Studies **60**
  Allocation Concealment **62**
  Exceptions to the Rule **62**
Sample Size **63**
  Which Formula? **64**
  Precision of Estimates **64**
Bounding Type I and Type II Errors **66**
  Equivalence **68**
  Software **68**
  Subsamples **69**
  Loss Adjustment **69**
Number of Treatment Sites **70**
Alternate Designs **70**
Taking Cost into Consideration **72**
For Further Information **73**

7 Exception Handling **75**
Patient Related **75**
  Missed Doses **75**
  Missed Appointments **75**
  Noncompliance **76**
  Adverse Reactions **76**
  Reporting Adverse Events **76**
  When Do You Crack the Code? **77**

    Investigator Related **77**
      Lagging Recruitment **77**
      Protocol Deviations **78**
      Site-Specific Problems **78**
      Closure **79**
      Intent to Treat **80**
    Is Your Planning Complete? **80**

PART II DO **81**

8 Documentation **83**
    Guidelines **84**
    Common Technical Document **84**
    Reporting Adverse Events **86**
    Initial Submission to the Regulatory Agency **87**
      Sponsor Data **88**
      Justifying the Study **88**
      Objectives **89**
      Patient Selection **89**
      Treatment Plan **90**
      Outcome Measures and Evaluation **90**
      Procedures **90**
      Clinical Follow-Up **90**
      Adverse Events **91**
      Data Management, Monitoring, Quality Control **91**
      Statistical Analysis **91**
      Investigator Responsibilities **92**
      Ethical and Regulatory Considerations **93**
      Study Committees **93**
      Appendixes **94**
    Sample Informed Consent Form **94**
    Procedures Manuals **95**
      Physician's Procedures Manual **96**
      Laboratory Guidelines **97**
    Interim Reports **97**
      Enrollment Report **98**
      Data in Hand **98**
      Adverse Event Report **99**
    Annotated Abstract **99**
    Final Reports(s) **102**

Regulatory Agency Submissions **102**
　　　e-Subs **104**
　　　Journal Articles **104**
　　For Further Information **105**

9　Recruiting and Retaining Patients and Physicians **107**
　　Selecting Your Clinical Sites **107**
　　Recruiting Physicians **108**
　　　Teaching Hospitals **109**
　　　Clinical Resource Centers **109**
　　　Look to Motivations **110**
　　　Physician Retention **111**
　　　Get the Trials in Motion **111**
　　Patient Recruitment **112**
　　　Factors in Recruitment **112**
　　　Importance of Planning **113**
　　　Ethical Considerations **114**
　　　Mass Recruiting **114**
　　　Patient Retention **115**
　　　Ongoing Efforts **116**
　　　Run-In Period **117**
　　Budgets and Expenditures **118**
　　For Further Information **118**

10　Computer-Assisted Data Entry **123**
　　Pre-Data Screen Development Checklist **124**
　　Develop the Data Entry Software **124**
　　　Avoid Predefined Groupings in Responses **126**
　　Screen Development **126**
　　　Radio Button **128**
　　　Pull-Down Menus **129**
　　　Type and Verify **129**
　　　When the Entries Are Completed **130**
　　　Audit Trail **132**
　　Electronic Data Capture **132**
　　Data Storage: CDISC Guidelines **133**
　　Testing **136**
　　　Formal Testing **137**
　　　Stress Testing **138**
　　Training **139**
　　　Reminder **139**

Support **140**
　　　Budgets and Expenditures **141**
　　　For Further Information **141**

11 Data Management 143
　　　Options **143**
　　　　　Flat Files **143**
　　　　　Hierarchical Databases **145**
　　　　　Network Database Model **146**
　　　　　Relational Database Model **146**
　　　　　Which Database Model? **149**
　　　　　Object-Oriented Databases **150**
　　　Clients and Servers **150**
　　　　　One Size Does Not Fit All **151**
　　　Combining Multiple Databases **151**
　　　A Recipe for Disaster **152**
　　　　　Transferring Data **154**
　　　Quality Assurance and Security **155**
　　　　　Maintaining Patient Confidentiality **155**
　　　　　Access to Files **155**
　　　　　Maintaining an Audit Trail **157**
　　　　　Security **157**
　　　For Further Information **158**

12 Are You Ready? 161
　　　Pharmaceuticals/Devices **161**
　　　Software **162**
　　　Hardware **162**
　　　Documentation **162**
　　　Investigators **162**
　　　External Laboratories **163**
　　　Review Committees **163**
　　　Patients **163**
　　　Regulatory Agency **163**
　　　Test Phase **163**

13 Monitoring the Trials 165
　　　Roles of the Monitors **165**
　　　Before the Trials Begin **167**
　　　Kick-Off Meetings **168**
　　　Duties During Trial **169**
　　　　　Site Visits **169**

    Between Visits **170**
    Other Duties **173**
  Maintaining Physician Interest in Lengthy Trials **173**

14 Managing the Trials 175
  Recruitment **176**
  Supplies **176**
  Late and Incomplete Forms **176**
  Dropouts and Withdrawals **178**
  Protocol Violations **178**
  Adverse Events **179**
  Quality Control **179**
  Visualize the Data **180**
  Roles of the Committees **183**
  Termination and Extension **184**
  Extending the Trials **186**
  Budgets and Expenditures **186**
  For Further Information **187**

15 Data Analysis 189
  Report Coverage **189**
  Understanding Data **190**
    Categories **190**
    Metric Data **192**
  Statistical Analysis **194**
    Categorical Data **196**
    Ordinal Data **197**
    Metric Data **198**
    An Example **199**
    Time-to-Event Data **200**
  Step By Step **203**
    The Study Population **203**
    Reporting Primary End Points **204**
    Exceptions **204**
    Adverse Events **207**
  Analytical Alternatives **207**
    When Statisticians Can't Agree **208**
    Testing for Equivalence **209**
    Simpson's Paradox **210**
    Estimating Precision **211**
  Bad Statistics **213**
    Using the Wrong Method **213**

       Deming Regression **213**
       Choosing the Most Favorable Statistic **214**
       Making Repeated Tests on the Same Data **214**
       Ad Hoc, Post Hoc Hypotheses **215**
   Interpretation **217**
   Documentation **218**
   For Further Information **219**
   A Practical Guide To Statistical Terminology **222**

PART III   CHECK   225

16 Check **227**
   Closure **227**
       Patient Care **227**
       Data **228**
       Spreading the News **228**
       Postmarket Surveillance **228**
   Budget **228**
   Controlling Expenditures **229**
   Process Review Committee **229**
   Trial Review Committee **230**
   Investigatory Drug or Device **230**
       Interactions **232**
       Adverse Events **232**
   Collateral Studies **233**
   Future Studies **234**
   For Further Information **234**

Appendix Software **237**
   Choices **237**
       All In One **237**
       Almost All In One **238**
       Project Management **238**
   Data Entry **239**
       Handheld Devices **239**
       Touch Screen **239**
       Speech Recognition **239**
       e-CRFs **240**
       Do It Yourself **240**
       Data Collection Via the Web **240**

    Preparing the Common Technical Document **241**
  Data Management **241**
  Data Entry and Data Management **242**
    Small-Scale Clinical Studies **242**
    Clinical Database Managers **242**
  Data Analysis **243**
  Utilities **244**
    Sample Size Determination **244**
    Screen Capture **245**
    Data Conversion **245**

Author Index 247
Subject Index 251

Chapter 1
Cut Costs and Increase Profits

THE ESSENCE OF THE GUIDELINES presented here—start with your reports, enter the data directly into the computer, validate on entry, and monitor your results continuously—first appeared in a newsletter I edited in the mid-1980s. The reactions of readers then ranged from tepid to outwardly hostile: "We can't afford to give every physician a computer," raged one data manager, ignoring the $10,000 per patient that is the normal minimal expense for clinical data. "What will become of all the people we've trained as encoders?" moaned another months before the furious downsizing that characterized the late '80s.

Such reactions make even less sense today when desktop computers are available for less than $1000 apiece (and are even lower priced when purchased 25 or 100 at a time), every corporation is leaner and meaner than it has ever been, and regulatory agencies around the globe actively solicit electronic submissions. Yet everywhere we look the same old-fashioned, outmoded, and hopelessly inefficient procedures are still in place.

NO EXCUSE FOR THE WASTAGE

There is no excuse for the wastage and only one explanation: Middle management in pharmaceutical and device companies have focused on their own survival, not the corporation's. They have minimized risks by doing what was done before and in consequence have placed the company at risk. They have developed elaborate time-consuming schemes to make today's paperless system function as though we still

---

A Manager's Guide to the Design and Conduct of Clinical Trials, by Phillip I. Good
Copyright ©2006 John Wiley & Sons, Inc.

had to carve out each letter by hand and cost their companies millions in unnecessary added costs and millions more in lost profits because of the delays.

And why the delays? So our manager won't rock the boat, be caught innovating, or, worse, bring on board persons with skills that fail to match existing job descriptions.

But the bottom line is that electronic data capture coupled with careful monitoring will cut costs and shorten the time to realizing profit.

FRONT-LOADED SOLUTION

This text is about a great deal more than computer-aided data entry. The essence of the solution is that we need to spend far more time on planning, less on the repairs.

My pessimism stems, in part, from my having spent the last twenty-five years as a consultant to drug and device firms. As a consultant, I was always called in at the last moment to "fix" the problem. The "fix" took months and was generally unsatisfactory, and all hope of profit vanished when the competitor was first to market.

I worked full time once, too, for a fast-track boss who'd earned his spurs as a firefighter. He put down every preventive measure I proposed. But then, what's a firefighter without a fire?

The solutions offered to you here are front-loaded and may seem expensive. But by putting in the preventive planning effort now, your company will avoid far more time-consuming and expensive delays later.

Anyone who has ever spent much time on the water (or in the air) knows that once underway it is far better to under- than to oversteer. On the other hand, no experienced sailor (or aviator) would consider getting underway without first making sure all systems were fully functional and life jackets, life raft, and emergency rations ready if needed.

I can understand and occasionally sympathize when biotech start-ups attempt to cut corners by doing the absolute minimum until they (and, more important, their investors) can

---

TWO APPROACHES TO MANAGEMENT

1. Tentative but responsible, avoids precipitous action and waits to see how the situation will develop before intervening.
2. Envisions the worst and plans for it.

Effective managers employ both.

be confident the project will be successful. It ends up costing these companies and their investors more in the end—not infrequently, an entire set of trials must be repeated all over from the beginning—but if you don't have money and must wait upon the necessary venture capital, what choice do you have?

The puzzle comes when a large well-capitalized firm makes the same errors, errors that can only be attributed to poor management and slothful minds that simply hope to defer the inevitable.

DOWNSIZING

Take downsizing as one example of sloppy management. Too often, downsizing has taken place by percentages and not in terms of the skills the modern corporation needs. Stand back, see what you are trying to accomplish, then hire, or, better still, retrain in accordance with current requirements.

Developing all the details of safety and efficacy assessment, data gathering, and recruitment before one begins demands time and patience. The counterargument that one cannot foresee every contingency is largely false. When one is forced to lay out all the elements of a design before commencing a study, one often manages to foresee 99.9% of the potential problems. Throwing up your hands and crying, "It's just too difficult, let's wait for the data," is the act of a child, not of a mature manager.

Often, those in upper management cannot understand the delay. Yet the tale of the ever-befuddled Bumbling Pharmaceutical and Device Company told in the chapters that follow is too often the case in all too many clinical studies. The high price of pharmaceuticals today masks the costs of ineptitude.

THINK TRANSNATIONAL

Once optimal dose levels and procedures have been established through Phase I and Phase II trials, begin to think on a transnational basis. Most large-scale trials are multicenter trials. By establishing your trial centers in several different countries, you'll have taken the first steps toward obtaining transnational approvals at no increase in costs.

The United States, Japan, and the European Union have already embraced the concept of the common technical document, simpli-

> Electronic data capture cuts costs and shortens the time to realizing profit.

fying the transnational submission process. The single set of standards makes it easier than ever to plan and coordinate your trials. And the transnational approach means an improved bottom line as your firm's new product reaches multiple markets simultaneously. It's good politics and can provide for more heterogeneous trial populations.

A FINAL WORD

For the vast majority of readers, no explanation of why we do clinical trials is necessary. Supervising or participating in clinical trials may even be your primary occupation. Still, there may be a few of you, inventors and entrepreneurs, who are asking just why your drug/device can't be marketed without expensive trials. It's been tested in the lab: You know it works.

The obvious reason is that the regulatory agency won't let you market your intervention without trials. But there is a greater, more important motivation:

Without an organized, well-controlled randomized clinical trial, a single run of bad luck, a whim of fate, could forever deny the public a promising cure and you and your company justified profits. Think of the controversy surrounding silicon implants. Women got sick, sued, and won millions in damages without the slightest scientific evidence supporting their claims. Manufacturers went bankrupt; hundreds of women had (as it proved, unnecessary) surgery to remove the implants. Yet these bankruptcies could have been avoided had the manufacturers of that period sponsored a well-controlled clinical trial.[1]

For your product to achieve the full success it deserves, you need to know what kind of individuals will respond best to the new treatment and what kind would do best to avoid it. Controlled large-scale clinical trials are the *only* way to get the answers you need.

> **IN THE NEWS**
>
> "German prosecutor launches probe against Bayer over how the company handled the withdrawal of Baycol/Lipobay, the anti-cholesterol drug that has been linked to fatal side effects."
> Financial Times, 4 September 2001. (In the litigious United States, just call 1-877-Toxic-RX to become part of a class action suit against Bayer.)
>
> "Baxter recalls blood filters after deaths."
> Financial Times, 4 September 2001.
>
> "Class action suit challenges Pfizer over the way it conducted clinical trials in Nigeria five years ago."
> Financial Times, 3 September 2001.

---

[1] Angell M (1996) *Science on Trial: The Clash of Medical Evidence and the Law*, New York: Norton.

> **CLINICAL TRIALS**
>
> Clinical trials consist of a randomized comparison over a fixed period of time of an intervention method (drug, device, or biological alteration) of interest against an established standard or a negative control (placebo).
>
> The trials are normally preceded by in numero (computer), in vitro (cell culture), and in vivo (animal) experiments, both acute (one time) and chronic (over an extended period), and, in some cases, retrospective studies of the effects of the intervention in humans.
>
> The initial Phase I or *safety trials* focus on the potential adverse effects of the intervention in humans. In the case of drugs and biologics, these trials are used to establish maximum acceptable dose levels (and the minimum toxic dose). They generally involve only a small number of subjects and a one-time or short-term intervention. An extended period of several months may be used for follow-up purposes.
>
> The subsequent Phase II or *efficacy trials* are used to establish minimum effective dose levels and to obtain some idea of the nature of secondary responses to the intervention and possible adverse side effects.
>
> The focus of this text is the final or Phase III clinical trial. These involve large numbers of subjects (500 to 5000), studied over an extended period of time (2 to 5 years) with the possibility of an even longer ongoing follow-up. The larger number of subjects in this type of trial provides an opportunity to study the effects of the intervention on different subgroups (women as well as men, smokers as well as nonsmokers, diabetics and nondiabetics) and to assess the effects of concurrent medications and various risk factors on the ultimate outcome. The longer time period provides for an assessment of the effects of chronic usage along with any other long-term effects.

Aspirin is unparalleled for its ability to ease pain, reduce fever, and suppress inflammations. I carry a couple of aspirin with me in the car because I've read that taking an aspirin during or just after a heart attack could save my life. But if I were already taking an anticoagulant, an aspirin could mean death.

On the back of the aspirin bottle, in large bold print, much larger than the other writing you'll find on the label, are the words, "It is especially important not to use aspirin during the last three months of pregnancy unless specifically directed to do so by a doctor because it may cause problems in the unborn child or complications during delivery." Important words that when written in the language of the potential consumer will forestall lawsuits.[2]

In what follows, we provide guidelines for your trials and a prescription for success. We tell you the contingencies you need to plan

---

[2]*Ramirez v. Plough, Inc.*, 6 Cal.4th 539.

for and the design decisions you need to make. We show you how to conduct and monitor long-term clinical trials and, finally, how to review the results so you can be still more effective in the trials of your next successful product.

Every profession likes to cloak its actions, even the simplest, in arcane language virtually unintelligible to outsiders (statisticians and computer scientists are particular offenders). We've tried our best to describe the work of the innumerable specialists in terms all can understand. Although I have many scholarly publications, my articles also have appeared in airline magazines, *Sports Now*, *Volleyball Monthly*, and a half-dozen newspapers. Hopefully, you'll understand everything I've written, the first time through.

I'd recommend you read this book twice, though: The first time to get an overview, and the second (and, perhaps, the third) time on a chapter-by-chapter basis as each stage in your trials arises. Each chapter contains checklists, so you might want to retain a copy of this book for yourself and put a second copy in the hands of the specialist who will be carrying out that chapter's functions.

Specialists (even statisticians and computer programmers) will also find this text of interest, not only for the checklists and lists of further readings that come with each chapter, but because this book covers and, hopefully, clarifies the activities of all the other members of the project team.

Thanks for reading.

Phillip Good, Ph.D.
Huntington Beach, CA USA
pigood@oco.net

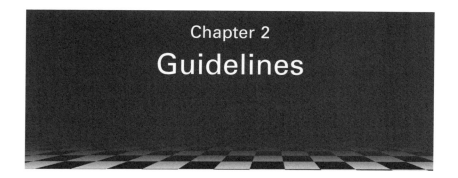

Chapter 2
Guidelines

THE PURPOSE OF THIS CHAPTER AND THIS TEXT is to provide you the manager with a set of guidelines for the successful design and conduct of clinical trials:

- **Start with your reports**
- **Keep it in the computer**
- **Don't push the river**
- **KISS**
- **Plug the holes as they arise**
- **Pay for results, not intentions**
- **Plan, do, check**

START WITH YOUR REPORTS

Let your objectives determine the data you will collect. Too often, data collection forms arise as the result of brainstorming by a committee. Ten questions on three forms for John's group and so forth (See sidebar.) The correct, effective way for study design is to list each of the study objectives, then backtrack to the data needed to perform the necessary calculations.

With price tags well into the millions, clinical studies today are not an academic exercise. The data to be collected should be determined by the objectives of the study and not the other way around.

Begin by printing out a copy of the final report(s) you would like to see:

A Manager's Guide to the Design and Conduct of Clinical Trials, by Phillip I. Good
Copyright ©2006 John Wiley & Sons, Inc.

> 743 patients self-administered our psyllium preparation twice a day over a three-month period. Changes in the Klozner-Murphy self-satisfaction scale over the course of treatment were compared with those of 722 patients who self-administered an equally foul-tasting but harmless preparation over the same time period.
>
> All patients in the study reported an increase in self-satisfaction, but the scores of those taking our preparation increased an average of 2.3 +1 0.5 points more than those in the control group.
>
> Adverse effects included . . .

These reports will determine the data you need to collect. Your list of potential adverse effects should be based on a review of past studies with your drug/device and with other agents in the same class of drug/device. In some instances, for example, when you want to demonstrate that your treatment is as efficacious as the standard but has fewer, less severe side effects, adverse effects should be a second or even a primary focus of your study.

Do not hesitate to write in exact numerical values for the anticipated outcomes, your best guesses. These guesstimates, for efficacy and for adverse effects, will be needed when determining sample size.

COLLECT ONLY THE DATA YOU NEED

"We need to cut costs," I was told by a group concerned with nicotine addiction. Could I help them develop a budget for a forthcoming feasibility study? They had ambitious plans. "We're going to collect the following data for each patient:

- Kansas Family Satisfaction Scale (4 questions)
- Motivation For Counseling Scale (24 questions)
- Internal Control Index (13 questions)
- Penn State Worry Questionnaire (14 questions)
- Nicotine Withdrawal Symptoms Scale (16 questions)
- Smoking and Prior Cessation History
- Vital signs including blood pressure, pulse, temperature, and respiration
- Laboratory results (electrolytes, hematology, creatinine, BUN, glucose fasting, pregnancy test results, and CO breath results)
- EKG findings."

I told them I was very impressed—we consultants lie a lot—then asked what they expected to include in their final report.

"The number of subjects that stopped smoking or reduced their smoking by 50%. And their withdrawal symptoms after six months."

"Will you be checking nicotine levels by urinalysis?"

"Can't afford it."

"You can't afford what you don't need either. And you don't need to collect data on anything other than a smoking and prior cessation history and the nicotine withdrawal symptoms scale."

We had our budget.

(See Chapter 6.) Make sure you've included all end points and all anticipated side effects in your hypothetical report. Once this prototype report is fleshed out, you'll know what data you need to collect and will not waste your company's time on unnecessary or redundant effort.

THE WRONG WAY

The wrong way to plan a study is to begin with the forms that were used in a previous set of trials. The sole reason for such a choice, regardless of all proffered rationalizations, is to shift the blame in case something goes wrong. The forms from a previous study seldom make even a good "starting point" (an often heard suggestion). Would you line up for the 100-meter hurdles where you stood to hurl the javelin? Never mind where the starting point used to be, locate the finish line, then back up 100 meters.

When and if you need to ask some of the same questions asked in a previous study, take advantage of your past experience to prepare questions that are unambiguous with definitions that exhaust all the possibilities.

KEEP IT IN THE COMPUTER

Enter your data into the computer and keep them there. Computerize:

- **Case report forms**
- **Laboratory instruments**
- **Data storage and retrieval**
- **Data analysis**
- **Report preparation**
- **Submissions**

Put a PC or computer terminal everywhere data are to be gathered. Computer-assisted data entry, that is, electronic data capture at the physician's workplace (hospital or office) and at the time of the patient's visit or procedure, simplifies forms design, speeds data entry, makes data entry less susceptible to error, and increases monitoring efficiency. Electronic case report forms are easier and faster to develop, as they eliminate time-consuming cutting, pasting, and renumbering, and facilitate last-minute changes.

Data entry can be via keyboard, touch-screen, voice recognition, or a hand-held device. As with ATMs, users can even choose the language in which the form may be viewed, facilitating multinational and multicultural trials.

Only a few regulatory agencies still require paper forms. Most prefer electronic submissions or e-Subs. If paper forms are required, they can easily be printed for signature afterward.[3]

From the study director's viewpoint, electronic case report forms offer at least four advantages over paper forms:

1. **Immediate detection and correction of errors**
2. **Reduced sources of error**
3. **Open-ended, readily modified forms**
4. **Early detection of trends and out-of-compliance sites**

It is well known that the ability to correct bad data declines exponentially with the time elapsed between the observation and the correction. By providing for validation of data at the time of entry, typographical and other errors can be trapped and corrected immediately.

Abnormal values (a blood pressure of 80 over 40, for example) would require confirmation at the time of entry or could be rejected altogether (like a BP of 12 over 8). Only subtle typographical errors would slip through—an 85 instead of an 86, but never an 85 instead of an 8.5. Missing values are forestalled.

Computer-assisted data entry means there are no intermediate forms—nothing is scrawled on the backs of envelopes or left to memory—nor are there errors in transcription, in copying and recopying.

Computer-assisted data entry facilitates monitoring and allows you to stay on top of problems. Once the data are in the computer, they can be collated back at your facility with data from other patients and examined for trends. If you detect ambiguities in questions or an over-used "other" category during the try-out phase, the electronic form is easily modified. You can also determine which sites, if any, may require additional assistance.

DON'T PUSH THE RIVER

More time is wasted by pharmaceutical and medical device firms in trying to fight, circumvent, or outwit government regulations, yet the regulatory agency's objectives are the same as yours: They want to

---

[3] In the United States, 21CFR Part11 provides for the use of electronic signatures.

protect the public from dangerous drugs and worthless devices; you want to detect and avoid problems before your products go to market and shield your firm from bottom line-destroying lawsuits.

This is not to say that one should abandon high-level intervention. In some countries (the United States is one example), prospects for regulatory approval may well be increased by hiring regulators as paid consultants or providing them with stock options.[4]

Still, time spent battling with a regulatory agency is time wasted, as is time spent on an inferior product. One fundamental rule should dominate your thinking: The quicker I bring a lawsuit-free product to market, the more money my firm makes.

Moral: it is better to anticipate and plan for regulatory agency objections than to try to circumvent them.

KISS

Keep it simple when you design your study, when you submit your protocol to the regulatory agency for approval, and when you prepare your reports.

Resist all temptation to use your study as a platform for experimentation, to compare alternate methods of measurement or alternate surgical procedures, unless such methods or procedures are the primary focus of and motivation for your study.

Simple, straightforward designs simplify training, encourage uniformity of execution, and are more likely to be adhered to in a uniform manner by your investigators.

Keep your intervention simple—a pill a day is preferable to three or four if you want to ensure patient compliance.

I hold little hope for a recently launched trial of a smoking cure that requires each subject to receive a preliminary three-day course of injections, take pills twice a day for ninety days, and attend weekly counseling sessions.

The same stress on simplicity should dominate your thinking when you set up time lines for the study. Follow-up examinations need to be scheduled on a sufficiently regular basis that you can forestall drop-outs and noncompliance, but not so frequently that study subjects (on whom the success of your study depends) will be annoyed.

---

[4]As reported by D. Willman in the *Los Angeles Times* for 7 December 2003, dozens of senior directors and researchers at the FDA received hundreds of thousands of dollars in consulting fees from firms whose drugs they were regulating.

Keeping your protocol simple will make it easier for the regulatory agency to grasp and provide fewer opportunities (handles) for objection.

The preceding rules go out the window when it is the regulatory agency that insists upon the complications (see, for example, Freedman et al., 1995). Ditto, if they ask for more data or more observations than you think is necessary. You can't control *them*. But, as they say in the psychology self-help manuals, you can control yourself.

Keep the forms simple—resist the temptation to ask redundant questions.

Store and retrieve character data in character form. "0" and "1" may have offered space-saving advantages in the '60s when a mini-computer might provide only four thousand characters (kilobytes) of memory and tape was used for mass storage, but today with even a personal computer's memory measured in millions of characters and compact disks holding billions of bits of information, you might just as well store "Y" or "yes" for yes as convert Y to a 1. (Or was a "2" a "yes"?)

Need to store the procedure name "atherectomy"? You could code atherectomy as a 411 or 502, but why not just as "ather"? As with all things simple, eliminating codes eliminates time-wasting coding and decoding as well as a major source of error. Plus, most regulatory agencies require the data in "decoded" format.

Keep the reports simple. If you, your employees, and your spouse don't understand them, regulatory agency reviewers won't either.

PLUG THE HOLES AS THEY ARISE

Computer-assisted data entry offers a tremendous opportunity for early detection of deleterious trends resulting from discrepancies in trial design or investigator inaction. It does, that is, *if* we pay attention to and act on the information we receive.

One of the earliest steps on the United States' path to putting a man on the moon involved putting a rhesus monkey into orbit. The monkey was watched and probed intently and studied from every angle. Evenings and weekends, in the absence of human observers, a dozen or more recorders kept track of the monkey's temperature, blood pressure, and other vital readings. Only no one looked at the output. The monkey was in orbit before the earthbound observers noticed he was running a fever. Yes, the monkey died.

A typical set of clinical trials today costs what that wasted space shot did in the 1950s. We needn't make the same mistakes that were made back then. Find the discrepancies and take advantage of the immediate availability of information that computer-assisted data entry provides to plug the holes as they arise.

PAY FOR RESULTS, NOT INTENTIONS

The most expensive single item in any study today is the physician's fee. Well, perhaps hospital charges can be appreciable as well. But you don't pay the hospital until after the surgery is completed and the patient discharged. Similarly, do not pay the physician (or specialty laboratories) until all the completed forms are in hand. (See sidebar, Chapter 14.)

PLAN, DO, THEN CHECK

Even if you follow every step of the prescription outlined in the next chapter, something is bound to go wrong or, at least, turn out differently from the way you anticipated. A study is never completed until you have reviewed the outcome, noted your errors, and, without assigning blame, prepared for the future. You'll find more on this topic in the final chapter of this text.

Part I
PLAN

We can't solve problems by using the same kind of
reasoning we used when we created them.
Albert Einstein

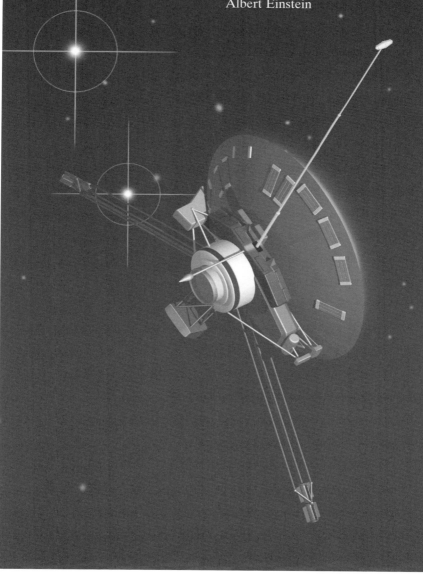

Chapter 3
Prescription for Success

THE PURPOSE OF THIS CHAPTER is to provide you with an outline of our prescription for success in the design and conduct of clinical trials.

PLAN

A. Predesign Phase

Form your design team (see Chapter 4). Your team's first step should be to decide whether the study is actually worth performing and whether you are ready to go forward.

Do you have the information you need on dosage, toxicity, and cross-reactions with other, commonly administered drugs? Are the details of any necessary surgical procedure(s) standardized and commonly agreed on?

Do you know which if any categories of patients should be excluded from the trials? Will the market for the drug/device/bioengineered formulation once these patients are excluded still justify performing the trials? And how many other studies on similar drugs, devices, or biologics are already in progress by competing firms? (See *http://clinicaltrials.gov/* for a partial answer to the last question.)

B. Design the Trials

Start with your reports. Let them determine the data you'll need.

Specify primary measures of efficacy. Decide what end points will be used to measure them. See Chapter 5.

A Manager's Guide to the Design and Conduct of Clinical Trials, by Phillip I. Good
Copyright ©2006 John Wiley & Sons, Inc.

> **EXCEPTIONS TO THE RULE**
>
> A full clinical trial may not be required. In the United States, "Any person seeking approval of a drug product that represents a modification of a listed drug . . . may . . . submit a 505(b)(2) application. This application need contain only that information needed to support the modification of the listed drug."[5]
>
> Applicants in the United States should submit a 505(b)(2) application if approval of an application will rely to any extent on published literature (as opposed to original clinical studies). This includes new chemical entities, new molecular entities, as well as changes to previously approved drugs. The latter category includes changes to dosage form, dose, dosing regime, or route of administration or even substitution of an active ingredient in a combination product.
>
> The FDA will accept a 505(b)(2) for a generic version of a biologic originally approved under an NDA. Examples include both naturally derived active ingredients and those derived from recombinant technology. Still, clinical studies will be required to demonstrate the similarity of the active ingredient(s) as well as a lack of immunogenicity.[6]
>
> "FDA may determine that manufacturers of biological products, including therapeutic biotechnology-derived products regulated as biologics or drugs, may make manufacturing changes (sources of raw material sources, production media composition, addition/removal/reworking of individual production steps, facilities, technology, and staff) without conducting additional clinical efficacy studies if comparability test data demonstrate to FDA that the product after the manufacturing change is safe, pure, potent/effective."[7]

Specify all measures of safety and any secondary measures of efficacy. Will you use checklists of adverse events at follow-up? Ask patients to volunteer concerns? Or do both? See Chapter 5.

Specify eligibility requirements. Too narrow a focus will force you to repeat the trials later and may make it difficult to recruit the necessary number of subjects. Too broad a patent may doom the success of the trials by including those unlikely to benefit from the intervention.

Specify baseline measures. Include all variables that might impact treatment outcome. (See Chapter 6)

Specify design parameters as defined in Chapter 6 including all of the following:

---

[5] 21 C.F.R. §314.54 [1994]
[6] If exclusivity is desired, additional clinical studies will need be performed.
[7] *FDA Guidance Concerning Demonstration of Comparability of Human Biological Products, Including Therapeutic Biotechnology-Derived Products*

- Treatment you will use with the control group
- Extent to which investigators will be permitted knowledge of the specific treatment each patient receives
- Whether you will utilize an intent–to–treat protocol
- Degree of confidence you wish to have in the final results
- Sample size required

Put your major effort into preparing for the trials, not in repairing them. Prepare for exceptions. See Chapter 7.

> Don't collect data you don't need.
>
> Store and analyze the data you do collect.

DO
Steps C–F can be executed in parallel.

C. Obtain Regulatory Agency Approval for the Trials
Obtaining regulatory agency approval can be as simple as submitting a written copy of the protocol you've already developed. (Government agencies being what they are, you may need to reformat the document to fit their requirements.) KISS is the operating phrase. Hopefully, simplicity was exercised in the design, along with clarity in writing the proposal. See Chapter 8.

D. Form the Implementation Team
Include a pharmacologist or manufacturing specialist who will be responsible for providing the necessary supplies. Allocate resources. Have your attorney review physician contracts. Hire documenters, lead programmer, and data manager.

E. Line Up Your Panel of Physicians
Don't underestimate the difficulty of recruiting and retaining patients. Decide how many clinical sites are required to recruit the number of patients you need at the time and for the duration you'll need them. Decide where to locate the sites. Would transnational trials be more efficient? See Chapter 9.

F. Develop the Data Entry Software
- Decide how you will collect the data.
- Decide what development software you will use.
- Prepare a time line for development and hire the necessary programming staff.
- Finalize the data to be collected. Determine the range of acceptable values for each individual data item.

- Develop data entry screens in sets corresponding to the individuals who will complete them.

See Chapter 10.

G. Test the Software
Conduct both automated and ad hoc tests, the latter employing individuals who will actually use the software. See Chapter 10.

Steps H–J can be done together.

H. Train
Three topics should be covered in a training program for the investigators and their staffs. See Chapter 10.

1. **Details of the intervention. The procedures manual developed in Chapter 8 will serve as text.**
2. **Data entry**
3. **Ensuring patient compliance**

I. Recruit Patients
Recruit patients and put in place measures to monitor and ensure patient compliance. See Chapter 9.

J. Set Up External Review Committees
The composition of these committees is considered in Chapter 4 and their functions in Chapters 4 and 14.

Steps K and L can be done together.

K. Conduct the Trials
- Review checklist, Chapter 12.
- Maintain a database and provide for its security. See Chapter 11.
- Maintain a schedule of regular visits to the investigators (in parallel with K). See Chapter 13.
- Collate data (in parallel with K). See Chapter 14.
- Prepare and review interim reports. Follow up on discrepancies and missing values immediately. See Chapter 14.
- Call meetings of the safety committee if necessitated by adverse event reports.
- Pay physicians and testing laboratories as completed reports are received.

L. Develop Suite of Programs for Use in Data Analysis
See Chapter 15.

M. Analyze and Interpret the Data
See Chapter 15.

CHECK
N. Complete the Submission
Prepare final report to regulatory agency. See Chapter 8.

Review study both to study weaknesses and to elicit findings that may serve as the basis for future studies. Prepare AAR. See Chapter 16.

Check with marketing regarding preparation of journal articles, physician guides, etc. Begin long-term follow-up and collection of postmarketing adverse event data.

Chapter 4
Staffing for Success

THE PEOPLE YOU NEED

Your first step in embarking on a new clinical study is to staff up to meet your needs. Although the natural temptation is to use those who assisted you in the past, a new approach may require new personnel with a different set of skills. The purpose of the present chapter is to list the personnel and associated skill sets you'll need to fulfill each step of the prescription outlined in Chapter 3.

Design Team

Given our emphasis on objectives, it should come as no surprise that the people you'll need most at the start of a project are those who will be present at the end to analyze and interpret the results.

I don't recommend the hiring of "design" experts unless they are experts at facilitating group discussions. Those who will reap are those who must sow. Nor do I advise your adding someone to the design team just because they are "available." To be effective, the members of the design team must be matched to the required skill sets that we cover at length below.

These individuals include the following:

The **project manager** whose chief skill is that of a facilitator, possessing the ability to draw out and motivate others, encourage differing points of view yet obtain consensus, assign and organize tasks, and make, not defer, decisions. He or she is responsible for establishing milestones, making personnel assignments, and tracking progress. Procrastinators need not apply.

A Manager's Guide to the Design and Conduct of Clinical Trials, by Phillip I. Good
Copyright ©2006 John Wiley & Sons, Inc.

Two physicians, one to concentrate on measures of efficacy, the other on adverse events. Both should be specialists in the area under investigation. As the two are intended to provide differing and, sometimes, conflicting points of view they cannot be in a mentor-student or a supervisor-employee relationship. Both will be expected to interpret final results and sign off on reports to the regulatory agencies. One or both will serve as **medical monitors** during the course of the trials.[8]

As discussed in Chapter 5, the two physicians will be expected to provide assistance in determining what information is to be collected and how measurements are to be made and interpreted. They will help in developing procedure manuals. They also will be expected to provide assistance and perhaps some direction in recruiting investigators for the study.

The medical monitors will answer all questions from investigators as to the procedures to be followed and will investigate possible protocol violations.

A **statistician**—preferably at the Ph.D. level. He or she will participate in the development of interim reports (see Chapters 8 and 14) and will supervise the final analysis.[9] In the design phase, she will be responsible for restatement of the design requirements in a form that lends itself to computerized analysis.[10]

One or more **clinical research monitors (CRMs)** who along with the medical monitor will serve as the principal points of contact with study investigators and their staff. They will participate in literally all phases of the study. Monitors must like to travel and be able to remain away from home for extended periods (they will have to remain in the field for training and perhaps to see the first several patients through the trial process at each site). They must have excellent communication skills and be able to maintain emotional as well as intellectual empathy with physicians and their assistants. The responsibility of maintaining morale over a lengthy trial process (see Chapter 13) often falls on their shoulders.

Monitors must also have an attention to detail. They need to have good speaking voices as they will be responsible for the training in data entry of the study physicians and their staff. During the design phase, they will be expected to acquire a knowledge of the clinical

---

[8] If not, a third physician, preferably one employed by your company, will need to be appointed as medical monitor.
[9] See Chapter 15 for a comprehensive description of these duties.
[10] See, for example, the section on determining sample size in Chapter 6.

trial literature for the specialty under investigation.[11] Obviously, their familiarity with past trials in the same area is a definite plus.

A **regulatory liaison**, who could be one of the above. The regulatory liaison's formal "role" is to interact with the regulatory agency, assuming (or, more accurately, sharing) the responsibility of interpreting the applicable regulations and ensuring that the trials remain in compliance.

A **marketing representative** can provide valuable input on desirable end points (you can't claim what you haven't established) and can aid in making the initial decision as to whether the trials are justified.

Obtain Regulatory Approval for the Trials

I highly recommend that a single individual make all primary contacts with the regulatory authority. At some point, a team physician may need to make contact with a physician employed by the regulatory agency or the team statistician with the regulatory statistician, but all such traffic should be arranged and directed by the regulatory liaison.

For preparing and reviewing submissions, the regulatory liaison should avail himself of the services of one or both of the physicians, the statistician, a medical writer, and the clinical monitors. He or she needn't be a gifted writer but should be able to direct the efforts of those who are. And the regulatory liaison needs to be a careful reader. Although all members of the team should be familiar with *ICH Guidelines on Good Clinical Practice*, it is this individual who must bear the responsibility for the final review.

The liaison should have the salesman's gift to "mirror" those with whom he's interacting. (Balance is essential and a hard sell definitely not advisable.)

Finally, he or she needs to have a positive attitude toward the regulatory agency. A need to outwit, circumvent, or simply oppose is a guaranteed recipe for disaster.

Track Progress

With the assignment of personnel to the team, begin to establish milestones and track progress. If multiple projects are underway, progress should be tracked across as well as within individual projects. A description of some of the available tracking software is provided in the Appendix.

---

[11]See, for example, the bibliography at the end of Chapter 5.

Implementation Team

Your implementation team will consist of a **pharmacologist and/or manufacturing specialist** who will be responsible for providing the drugs and/or devices needed for the trials; **clinical monitors** who will train, deliver, and monitor the ongoing process; **technical writers** to prepare the detailed procedure manuals for use by the investigators; the **lead software developer**, who will be responsible for developing the data entry screens as described in Chapter 10; and the **database manager**, who will be responsible for maintaining the integrity of the collected data as described in Chapter 11. The qualifications for the latter two individuals are outlined in the next section. You may also wish to add members whose primary concern is patient recruitment and retention.

Develop Data Entry Software

Responsibility for choosing the appropriate software for data entry, data management, and statistical analysis is normally divided among the lead software engineer, the data manager, and the statistician (subject, of course, to corporate approval, a topic on which we wax apoplectic in Chapter 10). The project leader may need to step in to resolve conflicts.

The **lead software developer** need not be a member of the programming team, but she must possess a general knowledge of both data entry and data management software and be able to prepare and maintain a flow or Gant chart for the development process. She bears overall responsibility for assembling the field specifications in collaboration with the clinical research monitor, and for approving the final screen designs. Ideally, she will also possess a knowledge of the statistical analysis software that will be used later on.

A team of Access or Oracle programmers will be needed to develop the data entry screens. They will not be working alone but in partnership with the clinical research monitors, who bear the responsibility for sequencing of questions and specifying the range of permissible answers. Programming sophistication is not as important as good interpersonal skills (particularly today, when the software does so much of the detail work). As illustrated in Chapter 10, a knowledge of ergonomics is essential.

The size of the team will depend upon the time lines that have been established. At least one member of the software design team should be from the testing group to ensure that quality is built in from the start.

Test the Software

Those who develop the software should no more be permitted to organize the final testing stages than a starting quarterback would be permitted to call defensive signals. For just as American football today has one team for offense and a second team for defense, so too should you have one team for development and one for testing: The two tasks require quite different mind-sets.

The testing team consists of one or more testing leads, the "formal" testing staff, and some "informal" testers. The **testing leads** are responsible for developing automated testing routines using such screen-capture utilities as WinRunner. (See the appendix on software selection.) Although the leads need to have a thorough understanding of the critical distinctions among unit, integration, and stress testing, the balance of the **formal testing team** can and ought to be relatively unskilled in computer use. Their task is to simulate the sort of errors that similarly unskilled personnel can make when the software is actually in use in the field. (Never mind that such "unskilled" personnel, physicians, nurses, and laboratory workers, may have solid credentials in noncomputer areas.)

I have found it useful to use one of the brighter new additions to the staff to serve as devil's advocate from the very beginning of the process. In the final stages of testing, the clinical research monitors, project leader, staff physicians, and other members of the design team should be invited to participate.

And don't forget the hardware. The testing team will need computers over and above the ones you already have. Those slated to go into the trial physicians' offices would be ideal. (Or, if these are sacrosanct, then additional equipment should be rented for the duration). You may also require additional support personnel to ensure that the testing team's computers will be up and running at all times.

> **DON'T FORGET THE HARDWARE**
>
> I once worked as a consultant to the team responsible for testing Xerox's ill-fated Globalview operating system. My job was to figure out why the group was falling behind. They'd doubled the number of testers, yet there was no corresponding increase in productivity. The not-particularly-complicated explanation was that the 12 testing personnel had been assigned only 3 computers, at least one of which was always unavailable while one or the other of the developers tried to figure out what had gone wrong.
>
> I'm sure Xerox's middle management already knew this; they just wanted the explanation to come from an outsider.
>
> Moral: Don't just hire people; create a working environment with all the software, hardware, and other tools these people will need.

Line Up Your Panel of Physicians

Putting together a panel of physicians and specialist laboratories is a nontrivial task to which (along with patient recruitment) we devote Chapter 9. Primary responsibility normally falls to one or the other of your lead physician investigators if he or she is an employee. Otherwise, recruitment becomes the project leader's responsibility. In either case, you may expect to require substantial assistance from the clinical monitors, who will need to inspect each site before approval is given.

An **attorney** is needed to draft contracts with the physicians and laboratories you've recruited. (See Chapter 7.)

External Laboratories

At issue is whether laboratory tests ought be performed in a centralized or decentralized fashion. The use of a single central laboratory not only offers the advantage of uniformity in measurement and measurement methods, but provides for more efficient and timely monitoring of results. To paraphrase Bernard Baruch regarding the stock market, "It's best to put all one's eggs in one basket, then watch the hell out of that basket."

Site Coordinators

Regardless of their prior experience with clinical trials, physicians invariably *underestimate* the amount of effort data collection will entail. Left to their own devices, physicians can and will assign supervision to overworked residents and nurses. The result, as one might expect, is both increased turnover of personnel and degradation in the quality of the data that is collected. The smart drug or device company will pay all or most of the salary of a *coordinator* at each site, thus ensuring both quality and continuity.

The coordinator, usually a nurse, is responsible for seeing that data is entered in a timely fashion and for ensuring prompt transmission of the data to the trial's sponsor. She will unpack the drugs and devices and verify that they are as requested. Often she will take on the responsibility of administering informed consent to the prospective patients. If not, she becomes responsible for seeing that informed consent is administered. If ambiguities arise or if problems occur in any aspect of the study (including the software and the hardware), she is responsible for notifying the clinical research monitor.[12]

---

[12]The presence of a site coordinator does not relieve the CRM of the necessity of making on-site inspections—see Chapter 14.

External Review Committees

You will need to establish several external committees whose members are independent of both your investigators and your staff to review trial findings. Each external committee will serve one of three main functions:

1. To review measures (e.g., X-rays, EEGs, ECGs, or angiograms) whose interpretation can be subjective
2. To determine whether adverse events should be deemed intervention related
3. To determine whether to continue or modify the trials based on interim findings

The committees appointed to review and interpret angiograms, X-rays, EEGs, and ECGs should consist of experts in the specific diagnostic area. The assignment-of-cause committee would consist of specialists in the disease process. The trial modification committee should include a statistician as well as physicians. All the committees should be able to call on additional experts—bioengineers, epidemiologists, geneticists, or pharmacologists—whenever they feel such services are warranted.

The primary duty of committee members is to ensure the safety of the participants in the trials. Their secondary responsibility is to ensure the integrity of the trials: the investigators, the regulatory agency, and the sponsor will rely on their advice. It is essential that membership be composed of individuals who are already recognized experts in their fields, and that these individuals lack any other direct connection with the sponsor of the trials.

The medical monitor will serve as liaison with all the committees.

Recruit and Enroll Patients

Without outside assistance, the typical panel physician may recruit as few as one-fifth of the patients he or she promised to deliver originally. Some may recruit none, taking their setup money and contributing nothing more, or recruit only one patient so that there is no offsetting control. We've outlined a number of techniques for increasing recruitment in Chapter 9. An experienced CRM could be placed in charge of the overall recruiting effort, aided by sponsor-paid site coordinators. Or you may find it more expedient to rely on the service of a professional recruiter. In any event, I would not recommend you wait "to see how the numbers turn out."

Transnational Trials

Effective execution of transnational trials requires that you designate a single coordinating center. This center will be responsible for

- Treatment allocation
- Monitoring of trial records
- Maintaining a central data depository
- Providing a home for field monitors (CRMs)
- Coordinating committees

In large-scale trials, supplementary regional coordinating centers may also prove of value to deal with potentially different rules, regulations, and cultural differences. See Williford et al. (2003) and Collins et al. (2003).

Conduct the Trials

Principal responsibility for the actual conduct of the trials rests with the project leader, database manager, and clinical research monitors. The latter's task is greatly simplified if you make use of paid study coordinators at each treatment site. The statistician may be needed to assist in the preparation of interim reports. Indeed, depending on the nature and duration of the study, virtually all members of the design and implementation teams may be called upon. In Chapter 14 we discuss the need to assemble **external review panels** and their recommended composition.

The project leader is responsible for authorizing payment to study physicians and other contract resource personnel (pharmacologists, radiologists, testing laboratories) as each individual milestone is completed. (See sidebar). Approval is generally pro forma once the clinical research monitors report completion.

The **database manager** has the continuing responsibility of seeing that the data are stored correctly, that their integrity maintained, and that they are readily retrievable. He or she is responsible for the integration of data from external sources—for example, from clinical laboratories. His or her knowledge must extend beyond an understanding of the data management software to security (maintaining onsite and offsite backups) and quality control.

Programs for Data Analysis

Development of programs for data analysis should be started on or before the actual beginning of the trials. One or more **statistical programmers** will work under the direction of the statistician. The ideal statistical programmer will also be a member of the team that develops the data entry screens. (Candidly, programmers who possess the dual set of skills are in extremely short supply.)

Analyze and Interpret the Data

Although the analysis is primarily the statistician's responsibility, he will need to work through the clinical research monitors and with the database managers to resolve any remaining issues of interpretation and data discrepancies. Clinical significance may be quite different from statistical significance (a point considered at length in Chapter 15); interpretation of trial results becomes the responsibility of the project leader drawing on the expertise of all the members of the design team.

THE PEOPLE YOU DON'T NEED

Too often throughout the '80s, and the '90s, and even today, downsizing was accomplished on an across-the-board percentage basis. Each

---

YOU DON'T NEED TO DO IT YOURSELF (BUT YOU PROBABLY SHOULD)

"The editors [of 13 leading medical journals] will criticize pharmaceuticals companies for their use of private, nonacademic research groups—called 'contract research organizations' (CROs) instead of scientists connected to universities and hospitals."
"CROs fail to provide sufficient oversight of clinical trials." from the *Financial Times* for 10 September 2001.

You can use your full-time employees to conduct the clinical trials or you can hire on a temporary basis a few or all of the people you need. You could have a staffing firm supply the programmers you need and place an advertisement for a consulting statistician. You can even hire a contract research organization (CRO) that will design and conduct part or all of the trials for you.

If you're a struggling one-product startup with just enough working capital, the lease versus purchase option can look awfully attractive.

Even well-established firms occasionally farm out their trials when they view their expanded needs as temporary or when a hiring freeze would make the trials impossible to conduct otherwise.

But a large firm doesn't just say to a CRO, "Here's some money, go do the trials, get back to me when you have the results." They establish milestones similar to those you encounter chapter by chapter in this text. An experienced full-time employee rides herd over the CRO's efforts. And even then, if complaints of the 13 medical journal editors are to be believed, such supervisory efforts are often inadequate.

Whether you decide to hire full-time employees, lease contract employees, or farm out the study to a CRO, you continue to bear the responsibility for the successful conduct and administration of the trials. Read on.

manager was given a quota, say 8%, to eliminate and then left to his or her own devices, a no-brainer that hardly justified the high incentives paid corporate cost cutters. True downsizing means reorganization and the redrawing of job descriptions to ensure effective performance.[13] In other words, someone who is not part of the design team and who will not be able to assist at other stages in the conduct of the study isn't needed any more. Put them to work elsewhere in the company, retrain them, or let them go.

More than one manager has told me, "If I do as you suggest and my head count drops below a certain number, then they're liable to let *me* go." If you're that manager's manager or, more aptly, the executive who dreamed up this absurd head count policy, do your company and your own stock options a favor: Resign.

Who Is on the Team?

	Number	Report to	Chief Roles
Project Leader (PL)	1		Facilitator, manager
Clinical Research Monitor (CRM)	1–2	PL	Liaison with investigators; assist PL with project administration
Site Coordinators	1 per site	CRM	Coordinate activities on site
Physicians	2		Determine data to be collected
Pharmacologist or Manufacturing Specialist	1		Prepare and deliver materials
Statistician	1		Determine sample size and methods of analysis
Regulatory Liaison	1		Liaison with regulatory agencies
Marketing Liaison	1		Needed during design/analysis
Attorney	1		Draft investigator contracts
Technical Writers			Prepare investigator manual
Lead Programmer (LP)	1		Develop data entry screens
Programmers	2+	LP	Develop data entry screens
Database Manager	1		Integrity and security of data

To say nothing of investigators, investigational laboratories, safety and efficacy review committees, and patients.

---

[13]Don't attribute this quote to me, Professor Deming and the pioneer industrial engineers of the 1920s said it long before.

FOR FURTHER INFORMATION

Collins JF; Martin S; Kent E; Liuni C; Garg R; Egan D; DIG Investigators. (2003) The use of regional coordinating centers in large clinical trials: the DIG trial. *Control Clin Trials* 24(6 Suppl):298S–305S.

Williford WO; Collins JF; Horney A; Kirk G; McSherry F; Spence E; Stinnett S; Howell CL; Garg R; Egan D; Yusuf S; on behalf of the DIG Investigators. (2003) The role of the data coordinating center in the DIG trial. *Control Clin Trials* 24(6 Suppl):S277–S288.

Chapter 5
Design Decisions

FROM THE OUTSET OF THE STUDY, we are confronted with the need to make a large number of decisions, including, not least, "Should the study be performed?" A clinical trial necessitates a large financial investment. Once we launch the trials, we can plan on tying up both our investment and the work product of several dozen individuals for at least the next two to six years. Planning pays.

Seven major design decisions that must and should be made before the trials begin are covered in the present chapter:

1. Should the study be performed?
2. Should the trials be transnational?
3. What are the study objectives?
4. What are the primary and secondary response variables?
5. How will the quality of the information be assured?
6. What types of patients will be included in the study?
7. What is the time line of the study?
8. How will the study be terminated?

> **PREDESIGN CHECKLIST**
>
> Before you can begin full-scale clinical trials, you need to establish:
>
> - Mutagenicity, carcinogenicity, and toxicity in animals
> - Mechanism of action in humans
> - Maximum tolerated dose
> - Minimum effective dose

Five somewhat more technical design decisions are covered in Chapter 6:

1. What experimental design will be utilized?

A Manager's Guide to the Design and Conduct of Clinical Trials, by Phillip I. Good
Copyright ©2006 John Wiley & Sons, Inc.

2. What baseline measurements will be made on each patient?
3. Will it be a single-blind or a double-blind study?
4. What sample size is necessary to detect the effect?
5. How many examination sites will we need?

Finally, we deal in Chapter 7 with the large number of minor details that must be thought through before we can conclude our preparations.

SHOULD THE STUDY BE PERFORMED?

We should always hesitate to undertake extensive trials when a surgical procedure is still in the experimental stages, or when the cross-effects with other commonly used drugs are not well understood. (A cholesterol-lowering agent might well interfere with a beta blocker, for example).

If your study team is still uncertain about the intervention's mode of action, it may be advisable to defer full-scale trials until a year or so in the future and perform instead a trial of more limited scope with a smaller, more narrowly defined study population. For example, you might limit your trial to male non-smokers between 20 and 40 who are not responding to current medications.

No full-scale long-term clinical trials of a drug should be attempted until you have first established both the maximum tolerable dose and the anticipated minimum effective dose. (In the United States, these are referred to as Phase I and Phase II clinical trials, respectively.) You should also have some ideas concerning the potential side effects.[14]

> **ONE TRIAL? OR MANY?**
>
> A single large-scale trial might appear more cost effective in the short term, says Michael Chernick of NNPI, but multiple tightly focused clinical trials generally are cleaner and faster. Multiple trials might be preferable in the following circumstances:
>
> - Testing for different disease conditions
> - Testing in different subpopulations
> - Testing for different effects
> - Monotherapy in one trial, combination therapy in another
> - Different control groups for one-on-one comparisons for different benefits
>
> The trials need not be concurrent and can often benefit from the results of other trials in their final design.

---

[14]See Fazzari, Heller, and Scher (2000).

SHOULD THE TRIALS BE TRANSNATIONAL?

If low incidence rates necessitate a multicenter trial, then active consideration should be given to basing the clinical sites in several countries. The United States, Japan, and the members of the European Community have all subscribed to the use of the Common Technical Document (see Chapter 8) in printed or electronic submissions. Not only does the transnational trial offer the advantage noted in Chapter 9 of diversified demographics, but it speeds and simplifies entry into diverse markets.

STUDY OBJECTIVES

I'm constantly amazed by the number of studies that proceed well into the clinical phase without any clear-cut statement of objectives. The executive committee has decreed "The intervention must be taken to market," and this decree is passed down the chain of command without a single middle manager bothering or daring to give the decree a precise written form.

Begin by stating your principal hypothesis such as

- **An increase in efficacy relative to X with no increase in side effects**
- **A decrease in side effects relative to X with no decline in efficacy**
- **No worse than but less costly than X and/or less invasive.**

X should be a positive control, an established treatment (whenever one exists) rather than a placebo.

For Motrin, the principal hypothesis was that Motrin would provide the same anti-inflammatory effects as aspirin without the intestinal bleeding that so often accompanies continued aspirin use.

The objectives of your study should be stated as precisely as possible. Consider the following: "The purpose of this trial is to demonstrate that X763 is as effective as aspirin in treating stress-induced headaches and has fewer side effects."

Not very precise, is it? Here is a somewhat more informative alternative: "The purpose of this trial is to demonstrate that in treating stress-induced headaches in adults a 5-grain tablet of X763 is as effective as two 5-grain tablets of aspirin and has fewer side effects." A marked improvement, though it is clear we still need to define what we mean by "effective."

A more general statement of objectives that may be used as template for your own studies takes the following form: "The purpose of this trial is to demonstrate that

- in treating conditions A, B, C
- with subjects having characteristics D, E, F
- an intervention of the form G
- is equivalent to/as effective as/as or more effective than an intervention of the form H
- and has fewer side effects."

Again, we still need to define what we mean by "effective" and to list some if not all of the side effects we hope to diminish or eliminate.

> **SET UP A DEFENSIVE TEAM**
>
> From the very start of the project, you need to establish a group whose primary purpose is to find the holes you have left in your design. I suggest a group rather than an individual, because in today's corporate environment, we all want to be thought of as team players. Moreover, not everyone makes an effective critic. If you are managing several projects simultaneously, then the members of one study group may be called on to criticize the efforts of the other. Otherwise, and in particular if your firm is a small one, it may be best to call on external consultants. Of course, your own role should be that of a facilitator rather than a proponent of any specific point of view.
>
> And, of course, at least one member of the review committee should have a copy of the current *ICH Good Clinical Practices* in hand.

END POINTS

Our next task is to determine the primary end points that will be used to assess efficacy. Here are a few guidelines:

- Objective criteria are always preferable to subjective criteria.
- True end points such as death or incidence of strokes should be employed rather than surrogate response variables such as tumor size or blood pressure. The latter are only appropriate (though not always avoidable) during the early stages of clinical investigation when trials are of short duration.
- The fewer the end points the better. A single end point is always to be preferred as it eliminates the possibility that different end points will point in different directions. On the other hand, as we shall see in Chapter 14 on data analysis, sometimes more effective use of the data can be made with a constellation of results.

The obvious exceptions are when a) surrogate end points are employed and a change in a single factor would not be conclusive; b) your marketing department hopes to make multiple claims; c) competing products already make multiple claims.

The end point can be determined in several ways:

1. **Duration of the symptom or disease**
2. **Severity of the symptom or disease at some fixed point after the start of treatment.** This latter can be expressed in terms of either a) a mean value or b) the proportion of individuals in the study

population whose severity lies below some predetermined fixed value.

For a blood pressure-lowering agent such as metoprolol, the primary end point is blood pressure. For an anti-inflammatory such as Motrin, it might be either the duration or the extent of the inflammation. For a coronary stenosis-reducing surgical procedure or device, it might be percentage of stenosis or the percentage of the population with less than 50% stenosis (termed binary restenosis).

An exact quantitative definition should be provided for each end point. You also will need to specify how the determination will be made and who will make it. Subjective? Objective? By the treating physician? Or by an independent testing laboratory? Is the baseline measurement to be made before or after surgery?

In a study of several devices for maintaining flow through coronary arteries, the surgeon who performed the operation made the initial determination of stenosis. But it was decided that the more accurate and "official" reading would be made from an angiogram by an independent laboratory.

How much give in dates is permitted?—patients have been known not to appear as scheduled for follow-up exams. What if a patient dies during the study or requires a further remedial operation? How is the end point of such a patient to be defined?

Don't put these decisions off for some later date; make them now and make them in writing lest you risk not collecting the data you will ultimately need.

Secondary End Points

Secondary[15] end points are used most often to appraise the *safety* of an intervention.

For a blood pressure-lowering agent like metoprolol these might include dizziness and diarrhea.

For an anti-inflammatory, the most frequent unwanted side effects are intestinal bleeding and ulcers. How does one detect and measure intestinal bleeding? Two ways: by self-evaluation and by measuring the amount of blood in the stool. Data relating to both must be collected.

---

[15]The use of the terms "primary" and "secondary" can be misleading. Quite often in long-term clinical trials, we are already confident in the efficacy of a treatment but are extending the duration of the trial so we can be equally certain of the absence of long-term negative effects.

> **END POINT OR SURROGATE?**
>
> I'm taking drugs currently to control my blood pressure and to lower my cholesterol. Thus my interests will be served if my diastolic blood pressure remains below 90 and my cholesterol dips below 200. Or will they? As my passion for ice cream reveals, I don't really care about cholesterol at all, or at least I didn't for most of my life. But I do not want to have a heart attack or a stroke, and I've been told that if I keep my blood pressure down and my cholesterol levels low I may well avoid both.
>
> It is both less time consuming and less expensive to measure changes in surrogate variables like cholesterol and blood pressure than it is to track survival. The former can be detected in days to weeks; the latter will (hopefully in my case) take many years. But can we always be sure that the surrogate variable we measure is directly related to the end point that is our real interest?
>
> Because very large-scale, very long-term clinical trials were conducted with government support, clinical trials employing surrogate variables such as cholesterol as end points are acceptable in some areas. But not in all. There are many documented reports of surrogate variables that have failed abysmally as predictors of sudden
> * cardiac death (CAST, 1989), cancer survival (Fleming, 1995), or AIDS recovery (Fleming, 1995).
>
> Any attempt to use a surrogate variable is sure to be viewed skeptically by the regulatory agency. It was not until well after the completion of LifeCore's clinical trials of its Intergel™ adhesion prevention solution that adhesion was declared to be an end point rather than a surrogate.
>
> On a further practical level, you cannot advertise what you do not demonstrate, and a failure to use actual end points will limit your subsequent marketing claims.

For a coronary stenosis-reducing surgical procedure or device, the primary concern is with other procedure- and condition-related adverse events including death, myocardial infarction, and restenosis severe enough to require further operations.

To ensure that you will collect all the data you need, a careful review of past clinical and preclinical experience with the present and related interventions is essential. For example, suppose that extremely high doses of your new agent result in the presence of abnormal blood cells in mice. Although such abnormal cells may be unlikely at the therapeutic dose you are using in the trials, to be on the safe side, blood tests should be incorporated in the follow-up procedure.

During the trials and after, you will probably want to record the frequency of all adverse events, of specific adverse events, and of those events directly related to the intervention that exceed a certain level of severity.

You should also determine *how* the adverse event data is to be collected. By use of a checklist—"Since your last appointment, did you experience fever? nausea? dizziness?" Or a volunteered response—"Have you had any problems since your last visit?" Elicited responses tend to yield a higher frequency of complaints. To be on the safe side both methods should be used. Of course, hospitalizations, emergency treatment, and phoned-in complaints between visits must always be recorded.

Some secondary end points may also be concerned with efficacy. For example, in a study of sedatives, you might be concerned with how rapidly the patient obtained relief.

> Don't Collect Data You Don't Need.
>
> Store and Analyze the Data You Do Collect.

Should We Proceed with a Full-Scale Trial?

The decision as to which changes in a primary or secondary end point will rule in favor of the null hypothesis and which in favor of the alternative needs to be made in advance of the trials for each of the end points. Nothing can be more embarrassing or useless than a large-scale trial that ends with signposts pointing in all directions (LRC Investigators, 1984). If the information needed to make these decisions is lacking, additional studies should be performed before proceeding with a full-scale trial.

Tertiary End Points

Tertiary end points such as costs may or may not be essential to your study. Don't collect data you don't need. When in doubt, let your marketing department be your guide.

Baseline Data

You will need to specify what baseline data should be gathered before the start of intervention and how it will be gathered—by interview, questionnaire, physical examination, specialized examinations (angiograms, ultrasound, MRI) and/or laboratory tests. Baseline data will be used both to determine eligibility and, as discussed in Chapter 6, to stratify the patients into more homogeneous subgroups.

Be comprehensive. Unexpected differences in outcome (or lack thereof) may be the result of differences in baseline variables. What isn't measured can't be accounted for.

Who Will Collect the Data?

One further step involves grouping the questions in accordance with the individual who will be entering the data, for example, demo-

> **CHECKLIST OF MEASUREMENTS**
>
> What is the nature of your intervention?
>   How will it be administered?
>   What is its duration?
> You are planning to test for efficacy.
>   What are your primary end points?
>   When will the measurements be made?
>   How will the measurements be made?
>   Who will make them?
>   What units will be used?
>   Who will interpret the measurements?
>   What quantitative results do you expect?
>
> You must test for safety.
>   What short-term side effects are expected?
>   How do you plan to measure them?
>   What quantitative results do you expect?
>   How soon can you expect to observe them?
>   What long-term side effects are expected?
>   How do you plan to measure them?
>   What quantitative results do you expect per 100 patients?

graphics and risk factors by the interview nurse with review by the physician, and laboratory results by the lab itself or by the individual who receives the report. These groupings will form the basis for programming the case report forms (see Chapter 10).

Finally, I would recommend that you charge specific individuals with the responsibility of addressing each of the points raised in the preceding sections. The design committee can then function as a committee should in reviewing work that has already been performed.

QUALITY CONTROL

The secret of successful clinical trials lies in maintaining the quality of the data you collect. The most frequent sources of error are the following:

- **Protocol deviations that result when the intervention is not performed/administered as specified**
- **Noncompliance of patients with the treatment regimen**
- **Improperly labeled formulations**
- **Improperly made observations**
    - **Inaccurate measuring devices**
    - **Inconsistent methods of observation, the result of**
        - **Ambiguous directions**
        - **Site-to-site variation**

- Time period-to-time period variation
  ○ Fraud (sometimes laziness, sometimes a misguided desire to please)
- Improperly entered data
- Improperly stored data

Among the more obvious preventive measures are the following:

1. Keep the intervention simple. I am currently serving as a statistician on a set of trials in which, over my loudest protests, each patient will receive injections for three days, self-administer a drug for six months, and attend first semiweekly and then weekly counseling sessions over the same period. How likely are these patients to comply?
2. Keep the experimental design simple; crossover trials and fractional factorials are strictly for use in Phases I and II (see Chapter 6).
3. Keep the data collected to a minimum.
4. Pretest all questionnaires to detect ambiguities.
5. Use computer-assisted data entry to catch and correct data entry errors as they are committed (see Chapter 10).
6. Ensure the integrity and security of the stored data (see Chapter 11).
7. Prepare highly detailed procedures manuals for the investigators and investigational laboratories to ensure uniformity in treatment and in measurement. Provide a training program for the investigators with the same end in mind. The manual should include precise written instructions for measuring each primary and secondary end point. It should also specify *how* the data are to be collected. For example, are data on current symptoms to be recorded by a member of the investigator's staff, or self-administered by the patient?
8. Monitor the data and the data collection process. Perform frequent on-site audits. In one series of exceptionally poorly done studies Weiss et al. (2000) uncovered the following flaws:
   - Disparity between the reviewed records and the data presented at two international meetings
   - No signed informed consent
   - No record of approval for the investigational therapy
   - Control regimen not as described in the protocol
9. Inspect the site where the drugs or devices are packaged; specify the allowable tolerances; repackage or relabel drugs at the pharmacy so that both the patient's name and the code number appear on the label; draw random samples from the delivered formulations and have these samples tested for potency at intervals by an independent laboratory.
10. Write and rewrite a patient manual to be given to each patient by his/her physician. Encourage and pay investigators to spend

quality time with each patient. Other measures for reducing dropouts and ensuring patient compliance are discussed in Chapter 9.

STUDY POPULATION

Your next immediate question is how broad a patent to claim. That is, for what group of patients and for what disease conditions do you feel your intervention is appropriate?

Too narrow a claim may force you to undertake a set of near-duplicate trials at a later date. Too broad a claim may result in withdrawal of the petition for regulatory approval simply because the treatment/device is inappropriate for one or more of the subgroups in the study (infants or pregnant women, for example). This decision must be made at the design stage.

Be sure to have in hand a list of potential contra-indications based on the drug's mechanism of action as well as a list of common medications with which yours might interact. For example, many lipid-lowering therapies are known to act via the liver, and individuals with active liver disease are specifically excluded from using them. Individuals using erythromycin or oral contraceptives might also have problems. If uncertain about your own procedure, check the package inserts of related therapies.

Eligibility requirements should be as loose as possible to ensure that an adequate number of individuals will be available during the proposed study period. Nonetheless, your requirements should exclude all individuals

- **Who might be harmed by the drug/device**
- **Who are not likely to comply with the protocol**
- **For whom the risks outweigh any possible benefits**

Obviously, there are other protocol-specific criteria such as concurrent medication that might call for exclusion of a specific patient.

Generally, the process of establishing eligibility requirements, like that of establishing the breadth of the claim, is one of give and take, the emphasis of the "give" being to recruit as many patients as possible, the "take" being based on the recognition that there is little point in recruiting patients into a study who are unlikely to make a positive contribution to the end result.

As well as making recruitment difficult—in many cases, a pool of 100 potential subjects may yield only 2 or 3 qualified participants—long lists of exclusions also reduce the possibility of examining treatment responses for heterogeneity, a fact that raises the issue of generalization of results. See, for example, Hutchins et al. (1999), Keith (2001), and Sateren et al. (2002).

In limiting your claims, be precise. Here are two examples: Age at the time of surgery must be less than 70 years. Exclude all those with diastolic blood pressure over 105 mmHg as measured on two occasions at least one week apart. (A less precise statement, such as "Exclude those with severe hypertension," is not adequate and would be a future source of confusion.)

Although your ultimate decision must, of necessity, be somewhat arbitrary, remember that a study may always be viewed as one of a series. Although it may not be possible to reach a final conclusion (at least one acceptable to the regulatory agency) until all the data are in, there may be sufficient evidence at an earlier stage to launch a second broader set of trials before the first set has ended.

> **BEGIN WITH YOUR REPORTS**
>
> Imagine you are doing a trial of cardiac interventions. A small proportion of patients have more than one diseased vessel. Would you:
> - Report the results for each vessel separately?
> - Report the results on a patient-by-patient basis, choosing one vessel as representative? Using the average of the results for the individual vessels?
> - Restrict the study to patients with only a single diseased epicardial vessel?

TIMING

Your next step is to prepare a time line for your trials as shown in Figure 5.1, noting the intervals between the following events:

- **Determination of eligibility**
- **Baseline measurement**
- **Treatment assignment**
- **Beginning of intervention**
- **Release from hospital (if applicable)**
- **First and subsequent follow-ups**
- **Termination**

Baseline observations that could be used to stratify the patient population should be taken at the time of the initial eligibility exam.

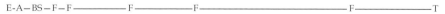

FIGURE 5.1 Trial Time Line Example. E eligibility determination and initial baseline measurements; A assignment to treatment; B baseline measurements; S start of intervention; F follow up exam; T final follow-up exam and termination of trial. Time scale in weeks.

(See Chapter 6 for a more complete explanation.) The balance of the baseline measurements should be delayed until just before the beginning of intervention, lest there be a change in patients' behavior. Such changes are not uncommon, as patients, beginning to think of themselves as part of a study, tend to become more health conscious.

Follow-up examinations need to be scheduled on a sufficiently regular basis that you can forestall dropouts and noncompliance, but not so frequently that study subjects (on whom the success of your study depends) will be annoyed.

CLOSURE

You also need to decide now how you plan to bring closure to the trials. Will you follow each participant for a fixed period? Or will you terminate the follow-up of all participants on a single fixed date? What if midway through the trials, you realize your drug/device poses an unexpected risk to the patient? Or (hopefully) that your drug/device offers such advantages over the standard treatment that it would be unethical to continue to deny control patients the same advantages? We consider planned and unplanned closure in what follows.

Planned Closure

Enrollment can stretch out over a period of several months to several years. If each participant in a clinical trial is followed for a fixed period, the closeout phase will be a lengthy one, also. You'll run the risk that patients who are still in the study will break the treatment code. You'll be paying the fixed costs of extended monitoring even though there are fewer and fewer patients to justify the expenditure. And you'll still be obligated to track down each patient once all the data are in and analyzed in order for their physicians to give them a final briefing.

By having all trials terminate on a fixed date, you eliminate these disadvantages while gaining additional if limited information on long-term effects. The fixed date method is to be preferred in cases when the study requires a large number of treatment sites.

TABLE 5.1 Comparison of Closeout Policies

	Enrollment Phase	Closeout	Total
Fixed Term	9 months	12 months	21 months
Fixed Date	9 months	12–21 months	21 months

> **WHO WILL DO THE MONITORING?**
>
> Monitoring for quality control purposes will be performed by a member of your staff, as will monitoring for an unusual frequency of adverse events. But at certain intermediate points in the study, you may wish to crack the treatment code to see whether the study is progressing as you hoped. Cracking the code may also be mandated if there have been an unusual number of adverse events. If a member of your staff is to crack the code, she should be isolated from the investigators so as not to influence them with the findings. The CRM should not be permitted to crack the code for this very reason.
>
> One possibility is to have an independent panel make the initial and only review of the decoded data while the trials are in progress. Greenberg et al. (1967) and Fleming and DeMets (1993) have offered strong arguments for this approach, while Harrington et al. (1994) have provided equally strong arguments against.
>
> Our own view is that a member of your staff should perform the initial monitoring but that modification or termination of the trials should not take place until an independent panel has reviewed the findings. (Panel members would include experts in the field of investigation and a statistician.)

Unplanned Closure

A major advantage of computer-assisted direct data entry is that it facilitates obtaining early indications of the success or failure of the drug or device that is under test (see Chapter 14). Tumors regress, Alzheimer patients become and stay coherent, and six recipients of your new analgesic get severe stomach cramps. You crack the treatment code and determine that the results favor one treatment over the other. Or, perhaps, that there is so little difference between treatments that continuing the trials is no longer justifiable.[16] Establish an external review panel both to review findings and, at the planning stage and after, to establish formal criteria for trial termination.

One school of thought favors the decision that you continue the trials but modify your method of allocation to treatment. If the early results suggest that your treatment is by far superior, then 2/3 or even 3/4 of the patients admitted subsequently would receive your treatment, with a reduced number continuing to serve as controls. (See, for example, Wei et al., 1990.) Others would argue that continuing to deny the most effective treatment to *any* patient is unethical. The important thing is that you decide in advance of the trials the procedures you will follow should a situation like this arise.

---

[16]See Greene et al. (1992) for other possible decisions.

If you find it is your product that appears to be causing the stomach cramps, you'll want a thorough workup on each of the complaining patients. It might be that the cramps are the result of a concurrent medication; clearly, modifications to the protocol are in order. You would discontinue giving the trial medication to patients taking the concurrent medication but continue giving it to all others. You'd make the same sort of modification if you found that the negative results occurred only in women or in those living at high altitudes.

A study of cardiac arrhythmia suppression, in which a widely used but untested therapy was examined at last in a series of controlled (randomized, double-blind) sequential clinical trials provides an edifying example. The trials were designed to be terminated whenever efficacy was demonstrated or it became apparent that the drugs were ineffective, a one-sided trial in short. But when an independent Data and Safety Monitoring Board looked at the data, they found that of 730 patients randomized to the active therapy, 56 died, while of the

---

BEWARE OF HOLES IN THE INSTRUCTIONS

The instructions for Bumbling Pharmaceutical's latest set of trials seemed almost letter perfect. At least they were lengthy and complicated enough that they intimidated anyone who took the time to read them. Consider the following, for example:

"All patients will have follow-up angiography at 8 ± 0.5 months after their index procedure. Any symptomatic patient will have follow-up angiograms any time it is clinically indicated. In the event that repeat angiography demonstrates restenosis in association with objective evidence of recurrent ischemia between 0 and 6 months, that angiogram will be analyzed as the follow-up angiogram. An angiogram performed for any reason that doesn't show restenosis will qualify as a follow-up angiogram only if it is performed at least 4 months after the index intervention.

"In some cases, recurrent ischemia may develop within 14 days after the procedure. If angiography demonstrates a significant residual stenosis (>50%) and if further intervention is performed, the patient will still be included in the follow-up analyses that measure restenosis."

Now, that's comprehensive, isn't it? Just a couple of questions: If a patient doesn't show up for his 8-month follow-up exam but does appear at 6 months and 1 year, which angiogram should be used for the official reading? If a patient develops recurrent ischemia 14 days after the procedure and a further intervention is performed, do we reset the clock to 0 days?

Alas, these holes in the protocol were discovered by Bumbling's staff only *after* the data were in hand and they were midway through the final statistical analysis. Have someone who thinks like a programmer (or, better still, have a computer) review the protocol before it is finalized.

725 patients randomized to placebo there were 22 deaths (Greene, Roden, and Katz et al., 1992; Moore, 1995; Moye, 2000).

My advice: Set up an external review panel that can provide unbiased judgments.

BE DEFENSIVE. REVIEW, REWRITE, REVIEW AGAIN

The final step in the design process is to review your proposal with a critical eye. The object is to anticipate and, if possible, ward off external criticism. Members of your committee, worn out by the series of lengthy planning meetings, are usually all too willing to agree. It may be best to employ one or more reviewers who are not part of the study team. (See Chapter 8.)

Begin by reducing the protocol to written form so that gaps and errors may be readily identified. You'll need a written proposal to submit to the regulatory agency. As personnel come and go throughout the lengthy trial process, your written proposal may prove the sole uniting factor.

Lack of clarity in the protocol is one of the most frequent objections raised by review committees. Favalli et al. (2000) reviewed several dozen protocols looking for sources of inaccuracy. Problems in data management and a lack of clarity of the protocol and/or case report forms were the primary offenders. They pointed out that training and supervision of data managers, precision in writing protocols, standardization of the data entry process, and the use of a checklist for therapy data and treatment toxicities would have avoided many of these errors.

Reviewing a university group diabetes program study, Feinstein (1971) found at least six significant limitations:

1. **Failure to define critical terms, such as "congestive heart failure."** Are all the critical terms in your protocol defined? Or is there merely a mutual unvoiced and readily forgotten agreement as to their meaning? Leaving ambiguities to be resolved later runs the risk that you will choose to resolve the ambiguity one way and the regulatory agency another.
2. **Vague selection criteria.** Again, vagueness and ambiguity only create a basis for future disputes.
3. **Failure to obtain important baseline data.** You and your staff probably have exhausted your own resources in developing the initial list so that further brainstorming is unlikely to be productive. A search of the clinical literature is highly recommended and should be completed before you hire an additional consultant to review your proposal.

4. **Failure to obtain quality-of-life data during trial.** Your marketing department might have practical suggestions.
5. **Failure to standardize the protocol among sites.** Here is another reason for developing a detailed procedures manual. Begin now by documenting the efforts you will make through training and monitoring to ensure protocol adherence at each site.

Other frequently observed blunders include absence of concealment of allocation in so-called blind trials, lack of justification for nonblind trials, not using a treatment for the patients in the control group or using an ineffective (negative) control, inadequate information on statistical methods, not including sample size estimation, not establishing the rules for stopping the trial beforehand, and omitting the presentation of a baseline comparison of groups. These topics are covered in Chapter 6.

Feinstein's final criticism was that one of the treatments had been discontinued despite there being no predetermined stopping policy. If you're read and followed our advice earlier in this chapter, then you already have such a policy in place.

CHECKLIST FOR DESIGN

Stage I of the design phase is completed when you've established the following:

- **Objectives of the study**
- **Scope of the study**
- **Eligibility criteria**
- **Primary and secondary end points**
- **Baseline data to be collected from each patient**
- **Follow-up data to be collected from each patient**
- **Who will collect each data item**
- **Time line for the trials**

Stage II of the design phase is completed when you've done the following:

- **Determined how each data item is to be measured**
- **Determined how each data item is to be recorded**
- **Grouped the data items that are to be collected by the same individual at the same time (See Chapter 10.)**
- **Developed procedures for monitoring and maintaining the quality of the data**
- **Determined the necessary sample size and other aspects of the experimental design (See Chapter 6.)**

- Specified how exceptions to the protocol will be handled (See Chapter 7.)

BUDGETS AND EXPENDITURES

> Those who will not learn from the lessons of history will be forced to repeat them.

Begin now to track your expenditures. Assign a number to the project and have each individual who contributes to the design phase record the number of hours spent on it. (See Chapter 15.)

FOR FURTHER INFORMATION

A great many texts and journal articles offer advice on the design and analysis of clinical trials. We group them here into three categories:

1. General-purpose texts
2. Texts that focus on the conduct of trials in specific medical areas
3. Journal articles

General-Purpose Texts

Chow S-C; Liu J-P. (1998) *Design and Analysis of Clinical Trials: Concept and Methodologies*. New York: Wiley.

Cocchetto DM; Nardi RV. (1992) *Managing The Clinical Drug Development Process*. New York: Dekker.

Friedman LM; Furberg CD; DeMets DL. (1996) *Fundamentals Of Clinical Trials*, 3rd ed. St. Louis: Mosby.

Iber FL; Riley WA; and Murray PJ. (1987). *Conducting Clinical Trials*. New York: Plenum Medical Book.

Mulay M. (2001) *A Step-By-Step Guide To Clinical Trials*. Sudbury, MA: Jones and Bartlett.

Spilker B. (1991). *Guide to Clinical Trials*. New York: Raven.

Texts Focusing on Specific Clinical Areas

Fayers P; Hays R. eds. (2005) *Assessing Quality of Life in Clinical Trials: Methods and Practice*. Oxford University Press.

Goldman DP et al. (2000) *The Cost of Cancer Treatment Study's Design and Methods*. Santa Monica, CA: Rand.

Green S; Benedetti J; Crowley J. (2002) *Clinical Trials in Oncology*, 2nd ed. Boca Raton, FL: CRC.

Kertes PJ; Conway MD, eds. (1998) *Clinical Trials in Ophthalmology: A Summary and Practice Guide*. Baltimore: Williams & Wilkins.

Kloner RA; Birnbaum Y, eds. (1996) *Cardiovascular Trials Review*. Greenwich CT: Le Jacq Communications.

Max MB; Portenoy RK; Laska EM. (1991) *The Design of Analgesic Clinical Trials.* New York: Raven.

National Cancer Institute (1999) *Clinical Trials: A Blueprint for the Future.* Bethesda, MD: National Institutes of Health.

Paoletti LC; McInnes PM, eds. (1999) *Vaccines, from Concept to Clinic: A Guide to the Development and Clinical Testing of Vaccines for Human Use.* Boca Raton, FL: CRC.

Pitt B; Desmond J; Pocock S. (1997) *Clinical Trials In Cardiology.* Philadelphia: Saunders.

Prien RF; Robinson DS, eds. (1994) *Clinical Evaluation of Psychotropic Drugs: Principles and Guidelines/In Association with the NIMH and the ACNP.* New York: Raven.

Journal Articles

The following journal articles provide more detailed analyses and background of some of the points considered in this chapter.

CAST (Cardiac Arrhythmia Suppression Trial) (1989) Investigators preliminary report: effect of encainmide and flecanide on mortality in a randomized trial of arythmic suppression after myocardial infarction. *N Engl J Med* 321:406–412.

Chilcott J; Brennan A; Booth A; Karnon J; Tappenden P. The role of modelling in prioritising and planning clinical trials. *http://www.ncchta.org/fullmono/mon723.pdf.*

D'Agostino RB Sr; Massaro JM. (2004) New developments in medical clinical trials. *J Dent Res* 83: Spec No C:C18–24.

Ebi O. (1997) Implementation of new Japanese GCP and the quality of clinical trials—from the standpoint of the pharmaceutical industry. *Gan To Kagaku Ryoho* 24:1883–1891.

Favalli G; Vermorken JB; Vantongelen K; Renard J; Van Oosterom AT; Pecorelli S. (2000) Quality control in multicentric clinical trials. An experience of the EORTC Gynecological Cancer Cooperative Group. *Eur J Cancer* 36:1125–1133.

Fazzari M; Heller G; Scher HI. (2000) The phase II/III transition. Toward the proof of efficacy in cancer clinical trials. *Control Clin Trials* 21:360–368.

Fleming TR. (1995) Surrogate markers in AIDS and cancer trials. *Stat Med* 13:1423–1435.

Fleming T; DeMets DL. (1993) Monitoring of clinical trials: issues and recommendations. *Control Clin Trials* 14:183–197.

Greenberg B. et al. (1988) A report from the heart special project committee to the National Advisory Council, May 1967. *Control Clin Trials* 9:137–148.

Greene HL; Roden DM; Katz RJ et al. (1992) The Cardiac Arrhythmia Suppression Trial: first CAST . . . then CAST II. *J Am Coll Cardiol* 19:894–898.

Harrington D; Crowley J; George SL; Pajak T; Redmond C; Wieand HS. (1994) The case against independent monitoring committees. *Statist Med* 13:1411–1414.

Hutchins LF; Unger JM; Crowley JJ; Coltman CA Jr; Albain KS. (1999). Underrepresentation of patients 65 years of age or older in cancer-treatment trials. *N Engl J Med* 341:2061–2067.

Keith SJ. (2001) Evaluating characteristics of patient selection and dropout rates. *J Clin Psychiatry* 62 Suppl 9:11–14; discussion 15–16.

LRC Investigators (1984) The Lipid Research Clinical Coronary Primary Prevention trial results. *JAMA* 25:351–374.

Maschio G; Oldrizzi L. (2000) Dietary therapy in chronic renal failure. (A comedy of errors). *J Nephrol* 13 Suppl 3:S1–S6.

Migrino RQ; Topol EJ; Heart Protection Study (2003). A matter of life and death? The Heart Protection Study and protection of clinical trial participants. *Control Clin Trials* 24:501–505; 585–588.

Moore T. (1995). *Deadly Medicine: Why Tens of Thousands of Heart Patients Died in America's Worst Drug Disaster.* Simon & Schuster.

Moye LA. (2000) *Statistical Reasoning in Medicine: The Intuitive P-Value Primer.* New York: Springer.

Sateren WB; Trimble EL; Abrams J; Brawley O; Breen N; Ford L; McCabe M; Kaplan R; Smith M; Ungerleider R; Christian MC. (2002) How sociodemographics, presence of oncology specialists, and hospital cancer programs affect accrual to cancer treatment trials. *J Clin Oncol* 20:2109–2117.

Weiss RB; Rifkin RM; Stewart FM; Theriault RL; Williams LA; Herman AA; Beveridge RA. (2000) High-dose chemotherapy for high-risk primary breast cancer: an on-site review of the Bezwoda study. *Lancet* 355:999–1003.

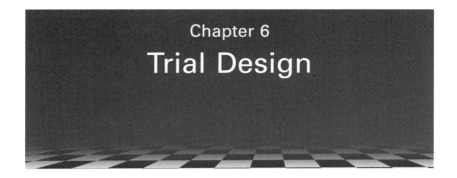

Chapter 6
Trial Design

ANYONE WHO SPENDS ANY TIME IN A SCHOOLROOM, as a parent or as a child, becomes aware of the vast differences among individuals. My most distinct memories are of how large the girls were in the third grade (ever been beaten up by a girl?) and the trepidation I felt on the playground whenever we chose teams (not right field again!). Much later, in my college days, I was to discover there were many individuals capable of devouring larger quantities of alcohol than I without noticeable effect. And a few, very few others, whom I could drink under the table.

Whether or not you imbibe, I'm sure you've had the opportunity to observe the effects of alcohol on other people. Some individuals take a single drink and their nose turns red. Others can't seem to take just one drink.

The majority of effort in *experimental design* is devoted to finding ways in which this variation from individual to individual won't swamp or mask the variation that results from differences in treatment. These same design techniques apply to the variation in result that stems from the physician who treats one individual being more knowledgeable, more experienced, more thorough, or simply more pleasant than the physician who treats another.

Statisticians have found three ways for coping with individual-to-individual and observer-to-observer variation:

1. *Controlling.* Making the environment for the study—the patients, the manner in which the treatment is administered, the manner in which the observations are obtained, the apparatus used to make

---

A Manager's Guide to the Design and Conduct of Clinical Trials, by Phillip I. Good
Copyright ©2006 John Wiley & Sons, Inc.

the measurements, and the criteria for interpretation—as uniform and homogeneous as possible.
2. *Blocking*. Stratifying the patient population into subgroups based on such factors as age, sex, race, and the severity of the condition and restricting comparisons to individuals who belong to the same subgroup.
3. *Randomizing*. Randomly assigning patients to treatment within each subgroup so that the innumerable factors that can neither be controlled nor observed directly are as likely to influence the outcome of one treatment as another.[17]

BASELINE MEASUREMENTS

In light of the preceding discussion, it is easy to see that baseline measurements offer two opportunities for reducing person-to-person variation.

First, some components of the baseline measurements such as demographics and risk factors can be used for forming subgroups or strata for analysis.

Second, obtaining a baseline measurement allows us to use each individual as his own control. Without a baseline measurement, we would be forced to base our comparisons on the final reading of the primary response variable alone.

Let's suppose this response variable is blood pressure. It might be that an untreated individual has a final diastolic reading of 90 mmHg whereas an individual treated with our new product has a reading of 95 mmHg. It doesn't look good for our new product. But what if I told you the first individual had a baseline reading of 100 mmHg, whereas the second had a baseline of 120 mmHg. Comparing the changes that take place as a result of treatment, rather than just the final values, reveals in this hypothetical example that the untreated individual had a change of 10 mmHg, whereas the individual treated with our product experienced a far greater drop of 25 mmHg.

The initial values of the primary and secondary response variables should always be included in our baseline measurements. Other essential baseline measurements include any demographic, risk factor, or baseline reading (laboratory values, ECG or EEG readings) that can be used to group the subjects of our investigation into strata and reduce the individual-to-individual variation.

---

[17]See, for example, Moore et al. (1998) and Chapter 5 of Good (2005).

CONTROLLED RANDOMIZED CLINICAL TRIALS

The trial design we shall be most concerned with in the present volume is that of the long-term controlled randomized clinical trial. By *controlled* randomized clinical trial we mean a comparison of at least two treatment regimens, one of which is termed a control.

Generally, though not always, as many patients will be assigned to the control regimen as are assigned to the experimental regimen. This sounds expensive, and it is. You're guaranteed to double your costs because you have to examine twice as many patients as you would if you tested the experimental regimen alone. The use of controls also may sound unnecessary. Your intervention works, doesn't it?

But shit happens. You get the flu. You get a headache or the runs. You have a series of colds that blend one into the other until you can't remember the last time you were well. So you blame your silicon implants. Or you resolve to stop eating so much sugar. Or, if you're part of a clinical trial, you stop taking the drug.

It's then that as the sponsor of the trials you're grateful you included controls. Because when you examine the data you learn that as many of the control patients came down with the flu as those who were on the active drug. And those women without implants had exactly the same incidence of colds and headaches as those who had them.

Two types of controls exist: passive (negative) and active (positive).

A negative control or placebo in a drug trial may consist of innocuous filler, although the preparation itself should be matched in size, color, texture, and taste to that of the active preparation. A negative control would be your only option with disease conditions for which there is no existing "cure."

More often, there exists some standard remedy, such as aspirin for use as an anti-inflammatory, or metoprolol for use in alleviating hypertension. In such cases, you would want to demonstrate that your preparation or device is equivalent or superior to the existing standard by administering this active preparation to the patients in your control group. Barbui et al. (2000) and Djulbegovic et al. (2000) recommend that an active control always be employed. Barbui et al. (2000) insist that to protect the patient *only* an active control should be employed. Depending on your requirements and those of the regulatory agencies, one or both types of control may be needed. (See also *http://www.ahcpub.com/ahc_root_html/hot/archive/2003/ama062003.html.*)

Another point to keep in mind is that a placebo generally cannot be considered equivalent to no treatment. For example, a recent study compared arthroscopic knee debridement, arthroscopic lavage, and placebo (sham) surgery for osteoarthritis. In the sham surgery, only skin incisions and simulated debridement without insertion of the arthroscope were performed. The result was that neither of the intervention groups reported less pain or better function than the placebo group (Moseley et al., 2002). That is, in this controlled trial involving patients with osteoarthritis of the knee, the outcomes after arthroscopic lavage or arthroscopic debridement were no better than those after a placebo procedure. In consequence, arthroscopic knee surgeries for osteoarthritis are now in disrepute and tend not to be performed.

Let's reflect on the consequences of not using controls. Who knows (or will admit) what executive or executive committee at Dow Corning first decided it wasn't necessary to do experimental studies on silicon implants because such studies weren't mandated by government regulations? It's terrifying to realize the first epidemiological study of whether breast implants actually increase the risk of certain diseases and symptoms wasn't submitted for publication until 1994, whereas the first modern implants (Dow Corning's Silastic mammary prosthesis) were placed in 1962.[18]

It's terrifying because the first successful lawsuit in 1984 resulted in a jury award of $2 million! Award after award followed with the largest ever, more than $7 million, going to a woman whose symptoms had begun even before she received the implants.[19] Today, the data from the controlled randomized trials are finally in. The verdict—silicon implants have no adverse effects on the recipient. Now, tell this to the stockholders of the bankrupt Dow Corning.

Randomized Trials

By randomized trial, we mean one where the assignment of a patient to a treatment regimen is not made by the physician but is the result of the application of a chance device, a coin toss, a throw of a die, or, these days, the computer program your statistician uses to produce a series of random numbers.

It may seem odd to circumvent the wisdom and experience of a trained physician in this way. Recall that the reason we are conducting trials is that we cannot yet state with assurance and government approval that one treatment regimen is better than another. Until our

---
[18] According to Marcia Angell (1996), the recipient of the original implants still has them and has no complaints.
[19] *Hopkins v. Dow Corning Corp*, 33 F.3d 1116 (9th Cir. 1994).

trials are completed and the data analyzed, there is no rational basis for other than a random assignment.

Warning: An investigator who has strong feelings for or against a particular regimen may not be an appropriate choice to work with you on a clinical trial. (See sidebar and Chapter 9.)

Blocked Randomization

Randomization means assigning treatment via a chance device. It does not mean giving the first patient the active treatment, the second the control, and so forth. A weakness with this latter approach you may have experienced yourself, on the occasional visit to Los Angeles, Atlantic City, or Monte Carlo, is that sometimes red comes up seven times in a row or you experience an equally long streak with the dice.

In the long run, everything may even out, but in the short run a preponderance of the subjects could get the active treatment, or in a multisite trial, one of the sites might have only control subjects assigned to it. In the first instance, a month-long epidemic of influenza could confound the effects of the epidemic with that of the

---

BIAS

Do we really need to assign treatment to patients at random?

In the very first set of clinical data that was brought to me for statistical analysis, a young surgeon described the problems he was having with his chief of surgery. "I've developed a new method for giving arteriograms which I feel can cut down on the necessity for repeated amputations. But my chief will only let me try out my technique on patients he feels are hopeless. Will this affect my results?" It would, and it did. Patients examined by the new method had a very poor recovery rate. But then, the only patients who'd been examined by the new method were those with a poor prognosis. The young surgeon realized he would not be able to test his theory until he was able to assign patients to treatment at random.

Not incidentally, it took us three more tries until we got this particular experiment right. In our next attempt, the chief of surgery—Mark Craig of St. Eligius in Boston—announced he would do the "random" assignments. He finally was persuaded to let me make the assignment by using a table of random numbers. But then he announced that he, and not the younger surgeon, would perform the operations on the patients examined by the traditional method to "make sure they were done right." Of course, this turned a comparison of surgical methodologies into a comparison of surgeons and intent.

In the end, we were able to create the ideal double-blind study. The young surgeon performed all the operations, but his chief determined the incision points after examining one or the other of the two types of arteriogram.

treatment. In the second, the aspects of treatment unique to that particular site would be confounded.

To prevent this happening, it is common to use a *block method of randomization*. The treatments are assigned a block of 8 or 16 patients at a time, so that exactly half the patients in each block receive the control treatment. The assignment to treatment within each block is still in random order, but runs of "bad" luck are less likely to affect the outcome of the trials.

Caution: Blocked randomization can introduce bias to the study. See Berger and Exner (1999) and Berger (2005).

Stratified Randomization

If you anticipate differences in the response to intervention or of males and females or of smokers and nonsmokers, or on the basis of some other important cofactor, then you will want to randomize separately within each of the distinct groups. The rationale is exactly the same as discussed in the preceding section: to ensure that in each group more or less equal numbers receive each treatment.

With life-threatening conditions the necessary data for stratification should be collected from each patient at the same time that eligibility is determined. This will permit assignment to treatment to be made as soon as eligibility is verified.

Checklist for the Design of a Randomized Trial

- **Always plan to conceal future allocations.**
- **Discuss openly the extent to which allocation concealment can be achieved.**
- **Carefully consider the patient population.**
- **Carefully consider the set of covariates to measure.**
- **Describe how prognostic each covariate is expected to be, and rank the covariates.**
- **Carefully consider the maximum tolerated imbalance.**
- **Carefully consider whether terminal balance is needed.**
- **Decide on the maximal, randomized blocks, or some other randomization procedure.**
- **Decide on the method, extent, and duration of blinding**

Source: Adapted with permission from John Wiley & Sons, Inc. from Table 8.1 of *Selection Bias and Covariate Imbalances in Randomized Clinical Trials* by Vance Berger (2005).

Single- vs. Double-Blind Studies

A placebo is a pill that looks and tastes like the real thing but has no active ingredients. It functions though the power of suggestion. The patient feels better solely because he thinks he ought to feel better. It will not be effective if the patient is aware it is a placebo. Nor is the patient likely to keep taking the drug on schedule if he or she is told that the pill she is taking morning and evening contains nothing of value. She is also less likely to report any improvement in her condition, feeling the doctor has done nothing for her. Vice versa, if a patient is informed she has the new treatment she may feel it necessary to "please the doctor" by reporting some diminishment in symptoms. These sorts of behavioral phenomena are precisely the reason why clinical trials *must* include a control.

A *double-blind* study, in which neither the physician nor the patient knows which treatment is received, is considered preferable to a *single-blind* study, in which only the patient is kept in the dark (Chalmers et al., 1983; Vickers et al., 1997; Ederer, 1975; Sacks et al., 1982; Simon, 1982).

Even if a physician has no strong feelings one way or the other concerning a treatment, she may tend to be less conscientious about examining patients she knows belong to the control group. She may have other unconscious feelings that influence her work with the patients. For this reason, you should also try to reduce or minimize contact between those members of your staff who are monitoring the outcome of the trials and those who have direct contact with the physician and her staff.

It is relatively easy (though occasionally challenging) to keep the patient from knowing which treatment she received. A near exception concerned trials of an early cholesterol-reducing agent, which had the consistency and taste of sand: The only solution was to make the control preparation equally nauseous. Not unexpectedly, both treatment and control groups experienced large numbers of dropouts; few patients actually completed the trials.

Keeping the physician in the dark can be virtually impossible in most device studies, particularly if it is the physician who performs the initial implantation. With drugs, most physicians can usually guess which patients are taking the active treatment, and this knowledge also may color their interpretation of adverse events.

A twofold solution recommends itself: First, whenever possible use an active control. A new anti-inflammatory should be compared to aspirin rather than placebo. Second, utilize two physicians per patient, one to administer the intervention and examine the patient, the second to observe and inspect collateral readings, such as angiograms, laboratory findings, and X rays that might reveal the treatment.

> **BREAKING THE CODE**
>
> An extreme example of how easy it can be to break the treatment code comes from a friend of mine who teaches at a medical school. He showed me a telegram he'd received from the company he was helping to conduct a clinical trial. They'd asked him to run an additional series of tests on half a dozen of the patients he'd been treating, including a PSA level. It didn't take a rocket scientist or my friend long to figure out that these had to be the patients who'd been given the drug under investigation. Not only had the trial sponsor broken the code by singling out some but not all of the patients for additional study, but they'd deliberately weighted the trials against their own product by failing to obtain an equal amount of adverse event data from the control population.

This last approach is often referred to as *triple blinding* in that neither the patient, the treating physician, nor the examining physician is aware of the treatment the patient receives.

In comparisons of surgical procedures or medical devices, a second physician should always be used. In a recent comparison of surgical procedures aimed at the reduction of postoperative pain, a physician independent of the operating surgeon issued all prescriptions for pain medication.

Allocation Concealment

It may not be possible to conceal the treatment from either the treating physician or the patient. But Schultz (1995) demonstrates that the treatment allocation must be concealed until the patient has been entered into the study. In other words, neither patient nor physician may have a role in the choice of treatment. And in a study of surgery vs. radiation vs. chemotherapy, for example, informed consent must embrace all three therapies.

Exceptions to the Rule

Are there exceptions to the rule? The regulatory agencies in some countries will permit variations from the fully randomized controlled long-term trial for certain highly politicized diseases (AIDS is a current example). But by going forward with such trials you run the risk that the results you obtain will be spurious and that after-market findings will fail to sustain or even contradict those obtained during the trials.

If you can't convince your boss of the risks the failure to use controls may entail, may I recommend a gift of Marsha Angell's 1996 book on the saga of silicon breast implants.

SAMPLE SIZE

Determining the optimal sample size is neither as complex as outlined in statistics textbooks—for there is ample commercially available computer software programmed to remember the details—or as simple—for the textbooks tend to omit too many real-world details. Eight steps are involved; fortunately, on an individual basis each step is quite easy to understand:

1. **Determining which formula to use**
2. **Collecting data to estimate precision**
3. **Setting bounds on the Type I and Type II errors**
4. **Deciding whether tests will be one-sided or two-sided**
5. **Letting the software make the initial calculation**
6. **Determining the ratio of the smallest subsample to the sample as a whole**
7. **Determining the expected numbers of dropouts, withdrawals, and noncompliant patients**
8. **Correcting the calculations**

INTENT TO TREAT

An obvious problem with a double-blind study is that it appears to rob the physician—the one closest to the patient—of any opportunity to adjust or alter the medication in accord with the needs of the patient. Thus many protocols provide for the physician to make an alteration when it is clearly in the patient's best interest.

Two policies preserve the integrity of the study even when such modification is permitted: First, the physician is not permitted to break the treatment code, lest she be tempted to extrapolate from the patient at hand to all those who received the same treatment. Second, the results from the patient whose treatment was modified continue to be analyzed as if that patient had remained part of the group to which he was originally assigned. Such assignment is termed "intent to treat" and should be specified as part of the original protocol.

As always, Bumbling Devices and Pharmaceutical carried the concept of "intent to treat" to an unwarranted extreme. At the onset of a single-blind study comparing two surgical procedures, a number of investigators performed the surgery first and only then looked at their instructions to see which modality ought to have been adopted. The result was a number of clear-cut protocol violations. (I place the blame for these violations not on the physicians but on the trials' sponsor for an inadequate training program.) Bumbling compounded their offenses and ensured total chaos by describing their study as "intent to treat" and reporting their results as if each patient had actually received the treatment she'd been assigned originally. One can only speculate as to the kind of penalties the regulatory agency ultimately imposed.

Which Formula?
We can expect to collect three types of data, each entailing a different method of sample determination:

1. **Dichotomous data such as yes v. no, stenosis greater or less than or equal to 50%, and got better or got worse**
2. **Categorical data (sometimes ordered and sometimes not) as we would see, for example, in a table of adverse events by type against treatment**
3. **Data such as laboratory values and blood pressure that are measured on a continuous metric scale**

We should also distinguish "time-till-event" data (time till recovery, time till first reoccurrence), which, though metric, requires somewhat different methods.

From the point of view of reducing sample size, it is always better to work with metric data than categorical variables, and to work with multiple categories as opposed to just two. Even if you decide later to group categories, income brackets, for example, it is always better to collect the data on a continuous scale (see sidebar). Some fine-tuning may still be necessary to determine which formula to use, but that's what statisticians are for.

Precision of Estimates
To determine the precision of our estimates for dichotomous and categorical data, we need to know the anticipated proportions in each category. As an example, if our primary end point were binary restenosis we would need to know the expected restenosis rate. We would need such estimates for both control and treated populations.

COLLECT EXACT VALUES

At the beginning of a long-term study of buying patterns in New South Wales it was decided to group the incomes of survey subjects into categories; under $20,000, $20,000 to $30,000, and so forth. Six years of steady inflation later and the organizers of the study realized that all the categories had to be adjusted. An income of $21,000 at the start of the study would only purchase $18,000 worth of goods and housing at the end. The problem was that those surveyed toward the end had filled out forms with exactly the same income categories. Had income been tabulated to the nearest dollar, it would have been easy enough to correct for increases in the cost of living and convert all responses to the same scale. But they hadn't. A precise and costly survey was now a matter of guesswork.

Moral: Collect exact values whenever possible. Worry about grouping them in categories later.

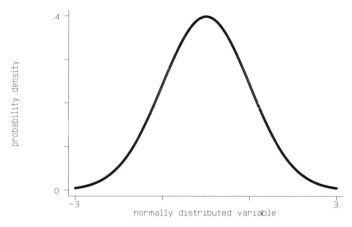

FIGURE 6.1 Bell-Shaped Symmetric Curve of a Normal Distribution.

Usually, we can collect data to estimate the former, but more often than not, we need to guesstimate the latter. One approach to guesstimating is to take the worst case, equal proportions of 50% in each treatment group, or, if there are multiple categories, to assume the data will be split evenly among the categories.

For metric data (other than time-till-event), it is common to assume a normal distribution and to use the standard deviation of the variable (if known, as it frequently is for laboratory values) in calculating the required sample size. You can see from Figure 6.1 that a normal distribution is symmetric about its mean and has a bell-like shape. Unfortunately, the distributions of many observations are far from symmetric (this is invariably the case with time-to-event data) and more often than not correspond to a mixture of populations—male and female, sensitive and less sensitive—whose distribution resembles that of Figure 6.2.

Too often, a normal distribution is used to estimate the necessary sample size, regardless of whether or not it is appropriate. If the data are unlikely to fall into a bell-shaped distribution, a bootstrap should be used to obtain the necessary estimate of sample size.[20]

When little is known about the potential magnitude of the effect, a two-stage or multi-stage procedure should be comtemplated. The

---

[20]See, for example, Manly (1992) and Tubridy et al. (1998). Details of the bootstrap method are given in Chapter 15.

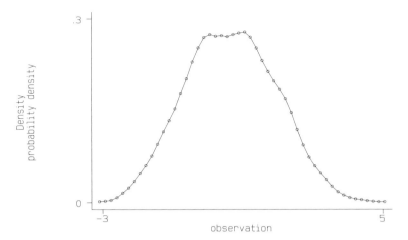

FIGURE 6.2 Mixture of Two Normal Distributions.

data gathered at the first stage should be used to obtain estimates both of the effect and of the variance in response, and, thus, to determine the size of the samples to be taken at subsequent stages. See, for example, Jennison and Turnbull (1999).

For time-till-event data, an exponential distribution or one of the chi-square distributions may be used to calculate the required sample size. See, also, Therneau and Grambsch (2000, p 61ff).

BOUNDING TYPE I AND TYPE II ERRORS

A *Type I error* is made whenever one rejects a true hypothesis in favor of a false alternative. The probability of making a Type I error in a series of statistical tests is called the *significance level*.[21] A *Type II error* is made whenever one fails to reject a false hypothesis. (See Table 6.1). When conducting a clinical trial, one can reduce but never eliminate these two errors.

Type I and Type II errors are interrelated. If we decrease the Type I error, by using a statistical test that is significant at the 1% rather than the 5% level, for example, then unless we increase the sample size our test will be less powerful and we are more likely to make a Type II error.

---

[21]The significance level should not be confused with the p-value, which is the probability under the hypothesis of obtaining a sample like the one in hand. The significance level is fixed in advance; the p-value is determined by the sample.

TABLE 6.1 Decision Making under Uncertainty

The Facts	Our Decision	
No difference	No difference	Drug is better
		Type I error Manufacturer misses opportunity for profit. Public denied access to effective treatment.
Drug is better	Type II error Manufacturer wastes money developing ineffective drug.	

The Type I and Type II errors, the treatment effect, and the sample size needed to limit the Type I and Type II errors to their predesignated values are all interrelated.

To detect smaller treatment effects, we will need more observations. We also will need more observations if we want fewer Type I or Type II errors. Consequently, to specify the required sample size, we first need to decide what size effect is really of interest to us, and what levels of Type I and Type II error can be tolerated.

Here is an example: Suppose that in 20% of patients, an untreated headache goes away within the hour. Do you want to demonstrate that your new headache remedy is successful in 21% of the cases? In 30%? In 50%? The less effective your new remedy is compared with the old, the larger the sample you will need to demonstrate a statistically significant improvement over the old.

You confront the same issues if your focus is on adverse events: The rarer the adverse event, the larger the sample you need to demonstrate a reduction.

Let's settle on the figure of 30% for the moment. (We can raise this figure later if we want to lower the sample size and feel sufficiently confident in our product to make the adjustment.) The maximum allowable Type I error is normally specified by the regulatory agency. For establishing a primary response, 5% is customary. The Type II error or, equivalently, the power,[22] is under our control.

How certain do you want to be of detecting the improvement your treatment offers? Fifty percent of the time? Hardly adequate, not

---

[22] The *power* of a test is defined as the complement of the probability of making a Type II error, that is, the probability of correctly rejecting a false hypothesis and accepting the alternative. The more powerful the test, the smaller the Type I error.

after you've spent several million dollars conducting the trials. Ninety percent? Ninety-five? Of course, you'd like to establish that there is a difference 100% of the time, but unless your remedy works in 100% of cases, it can't be done, at least not without an infinite number of patients.

In the end, the bound on Type II error you and your statistician arrive at may have to represent a compromise between how much you are willing to spend on the trials and how reluctant you are to let a promising remedy slip through your hands.

Warning: Changing the Type I error bound (the significance level) after the experiment is *not* acceptable; see Moye (1998; 2000, p. 149).

Equivalence

The preceding discussion is based on the premise that you want to show that your treatment represents an improvement over the old one. If instead you want to demonstrate equivalence,[23] then you may want to keep the sample size as small as possible. For as the sample grows larger and larger, you are guaranteed to reject the hypothesis of equivalence no matter how small the actual difference between the effects of the two treatments may be.

Whether you are testing that two treatments are equivalent or that one is superior to the other, a sample size that is adequate for establishing a treatment's *efficacy* may not be adequate for establishing its *safety*. More and more often, regulatory agencies are imposing a bound on the Type II errors allowable when reporting adverse events. The more rare and more severe the event, the larger the sample required to eliminate fears of its occurrence. In the end, the bound set by the regulatory agency rather than the needs of your firm may determine your sample size.

Software

We've listed some of the computer software that can be used for sample size calculations such as nQuery, Pass 2000, Power and Precision, S-PLUS, and StatXact in an Appendix. For additional details on the methods of calculation, see Shuster (1993).

---

[23]When we say two treatments are equivalent, we don't really mean they have identical effects, merely that they are sufficiently close in effect that physiologically they cannot be told apart.

Subsamples

The number the software's calculations yield may appear rather smaller than you expected. That's the good news. The bad news is that this number may represent only a small fraction of the sample you'll need to consider when all cofactors are taken into consideration. The worst case occurs when you expect to find differences in the magnitude (and perhaps even the direction, plus or minus) of the treatment effect depending on whether the subject is male or female, a smoker or nonsmoker, has multiple risk factors or none at all, and so forth. When you are almost certain such *interactions* don't exist (you can never be absolutely sure) then rather than double the total sample size, you may only need to increase it by one or two additional observations for each cofactor.

In the worst case scenario, you'll need to double the sample size you calculated initially to include both males and females, double it again to include smokers and nonsmokers, double it a third time to include treated subjects as well controls, and so on; the final result may be undesirably large.

Loss Adjustment

Alas, even this result is not final, for it represents only those subjects who will complete the study. You can expect to lose many patients along the way.

The greatest losses, sometimes exceeding 90%, occur during the initial screen. The cost to you of these ineligibles is thus a minimum; still, they have to be accounted for. Unfortunately, the clinical literature provides no consistent guidelines for determining the exact percentage of those interviewed who will go on to actually participate in the study.

Hopefully you can rely on the past experience of yourself and your colleagues. Don't hesitate to do what you can to improve the numbers—in Chapter 9, we discuss several methods for increasing the percentage you enroll—but you will need to multiply the numbers you came up with originally to correct for ineligibles.

The second set of losses occurs once the trials are under way as a result of dropouts and noncompliance. Patients don't remain on their medication, or begin to self-dose with some unrelated drug. Patients don't show up for appointments. Or patients may drop out of the trials altogether. In Chapters 9 and 12, we discuss methods you can employ to reduce these losses. Again, you must factor in these yet-to-occur losses before settling on a final figure for the size of the initial sample.

NUMBER OF TREATMENT SITES

If all the information you needed could be collected at a single site, the result would be an immediate reduction in patient-to-patient variation with an accompanying decrease in the necessary sample size. But that's not going to happen, particularly if the disease condition you hope to treat is a relatively rare one. Even if it could happen, you might want to use multiple sites if you felt it would reduce the total time required to complete the trials.

Either way you need to have some advance notion of the number of patients you might hope to treat at each site, which means you have to have some notion of the prevalence of the disease condition. If you come up with less than six patients per site, then you will need to increase the duration of your study in order to enroll sufficient eligible patients (see also Chapter 9).

Once you have this number in hand, you can divide the sample size by it to determine the number of physicians you will need to recruit.

> **PRACTICAL STEPS YOU CAN TAKE TO REDUCE LOSSES**
>
> - Target recruiting efforts at those both eligible and likely to participate (See Chapter 9).
> - Review and, if possible, loosen eligibility requirements.
> - Select appropriate participants, i.e., ones most likely to remain in compliance.
> - Establish measures to increase compliance (see Chapter 5).

ALTERNATE DESIGNS

KISS is the operative phrase in the design of the large-scale long-term randomized controlled clinical trials that are the chief concern of this volume. We advise you to resist all attempts to measure redundant variables ("But surely as long as the patient is in my office you won't mind if I perform one or two tests of my own?") or complicate the design. On the other hand, short-term clinical trials of more limited scope whose objective is to determine the maximum tolerable dose or to establish efficacy can often benefit from the use of more complex experimental designs such as a crossover or a fractional factorial.

In a *crossover design*, each patient receives all treatments in order, Treatment A followed by Treatment B, or Treatment B followed by Treatment A (or, if there are more alternatives, A followed by B followed by C). Thus each patient serves as her own control, reducing the individual-to-individual variance to an absolute minimum.

In a *fractional factorial design*, best employed when there are adjunct treatments and/or multiple cofactors, only some and not all treatment combinations are tested. Sophisticated statistical methods are used during the analysis phase to compensate for the missing data.

The advantage both these design types offer is that they markedly reduce the total number of patients required for the trials. Their disadvantage, again in both cases, is that their validity rests on certain key assumptions that are seldom realized in practice.

To use a crossover design, one has to assume that neither treatment has a residual effect, that using B after A has exactly the same effect on a patient as if A had never been used. In particular, one has to assume that trace quantities of A and its metabolic by-products do not linger in the body after treatment with A is ended. If crossover trials are contemplated, a pharmacokineticist is an essential addition to the design team.

To maintain the validity of a fractional factorial design one has to be able to assume that the effect of Treatment A is the same at all levels of the cofactor and in all subgroups. Again, these assumptions are seldom realized in practice and represent major drawbacks for the methodology.

But the main objection to these designs is that full-scale, long-term clinical trials have not one but two purposes: to demonstrate *both* efficacy and safety. A sample size that might be adequate for demonstrating the one may be far too small to establish the other. The chief advantage of crossover and fractional factorial designs—reduction in sample size—is lost, while their disadvantages remain.

A third type of study, occasionally used to demonstrate efficacy, employs *case controls*. The data for these controls are obtained by referencing historical databases and attempting to find patients whose profiles (demographics, risk factors, laboratory values) align as closely as possible with those of patients who received the investigational intervention. As the allocation of patients to treatment was not made at random, and the treatments of control and experimental subjects were not contemporaneous, this type of design is not appropriate for full-scale clinical trials. They can be useful in demonstrating to the regulatory agency the validity of going forward with large-scale clinical trials (see Chapter 8).

If death is a possible outcome for an untreated or inadequately treated patient as it is, for example, with AIDS, you may want to consider the use of *response adaptive randomization* in which the majority of new patients are assigned to the currently most successful treatment. If the "success" was temporary or merely a chance event, then the proportions will gradually even out again or perhaps go the other way. But if further trials sustain the advantages of one treatment over another, then a greater and greater proportion of patients will be assigned to the preferable treatment and the number of deaths during the trials will be kept to a minimum.

The analysis of such trials is complicated, but it is well understood and thoroughly documented; see for example, Yao and Wei (1996) and Li, Shih, and Wang (2005). The chief drawback until recently was the lack of commercially available software with which to design the experiment and perform the analysis. Fortunately, S+SeqTrial and EAST are now available (see Appendix).

TAKING COST INTO CONSIDERATION

The chief controllable factors affecting the cost of clinical trials are

- Choice of end points
- Data entry
- Eligibility criteria
- Patient recruiting methods
- Physician reimbursement
- Sample size
- Duration of the trials

Profit considerations should be taken into account when making decisions about the design of randomized controlled trials. For example, more precise measurements are generally more costly but their use can reduce the number of patients that are required. A cost analysis of all alternatives should be made before the final choice of end points is made.

Sample sizes need not be balanced. A design that assigns more patients to the less costly treatment group can be more cost effective; see, for example, Torgerson and Campbell (1997).

Computer-aided direct data entry will result in a substantial reduction in costs and, along with computer-aided NDAs, will increase profits by allowing you to bring a product to market sooner; see Chapters 8 and 10.

Chapter 9 contains a number of suggestions for making patient recruiting efforts more cost effective.

Economic models can be used to determine a portfolio of studies that maximizes the expected return on a given development or trial budget. See, for example, Backhouse (1998), Cavan (1995), and Claxton and Posnett (1996).

FOR FURTHER INFORMATION

Angell M. (1996) *Science on Trial: The Clash of Medical Evidence and the Law.* New York: Norton.

Backhouse ME. (1998) An investment appraisal approach to clinical trial design. *Health Econ* 7:605–619.

Barbui C; Violante A; Garattini S. (2000) Does placebo help establish equivalence in trials of new antidepressants? *Eur Psychiatry* 15:268–273.

Berger VW; Exner DV (1999) Detecting selection bias in randomized clinical trials. *Control Clin Trials* 20:319–327.

Berger VW. (2005) *Selection Bias and Covariate Imbalances in Randomized Clinical Trials.* Chichester: John Wiley & Sons.

Berlin JA; Ness RB. (1996) Randomized clinical-trials in the presence of diagnostic uncertainty—implications for measures of efficacy and sample-size. *Control Clin Trials* 17:191–200.

Cavan BN. (1995) Improving clinical trials cost management in biotech companies. *Biotechnology* (NY). 13:226–228.

Chalmers, TC; Celano P; Sacks HS; Smith H. (1983). Bias in treatment assignment in controlled clinical trials. *N Engl J Med* 309:1358–1361.

Claxton K; Posnett J. (1996) An economic approach to clinical trial design and research priority-setting. *Health Econ* 5:513–524.

Djulbegovic B; Lacevic M; Cantor A; Fields KK; Bennett CL; Adams JR; Kuderer NM; Lyman GH. (2000) The uncertainty principle and industry-sponsored research. *Lancet* 356:635–638.

Ederer F. (1975). Why do we need controls? Why do we need to randomize? *Am J Ophthalmol* 76:758–762.

Elwood JM. (1998) *Critical Appraisal Of Epidemiological Studies And Clinical Trials*, 2nd ed. New York: Oxford University Press.

Good PI. (2005) *Resampling Methods.* Boston: Birkhauser.

ICH (1998) E 9 Statistical Principles for Clinical Trials. *Federal Register* 63:49583. http://www.fda.gov/cder/guidance/91698.pdf.

ICH (2001) *E 10 Choice of Control Group and Related Issues in Clinical Trials.* http://www.fda.gov/cder/guidance/4155fnl.htm.

Jennison C; Turnbull BW. (1999) *Group Sequential Methods with Applications to Clinical Trials.* Chapman & Hall/CRC.

Jones B; Kenward MG. (1989) *Design and Analysis of Crossover Trials.* New York: Chapman and Hall.

Karlsson J; Engebretsen L; Dainty K; ISAKOS Scientific Committee. (2003) Considerations on sample size and power calculations in randomized clinical trials. *Arthroscopy* 19:997–999.

Li G; Shih WJ; Wang Y. (2005) Two-stage adaptive design for clinical trials with survival data. *J Biopharm Stat* 15:707–718.

Maggard MA; O'Connell JB; Liu JH; Etzioni DA; Ko CY. (2003) Sample size calculations in surgery: are they done correctly? *J Postgrad Med* 49:109–113.

Manly BFJ. (1992) Bootstrapping for determining sample sizes in biological studies. *J Exp Mar Biol Ecol* 158:189–196.

Matthews JNS. (2001) *An Introduction to Randomized Controlled Clinical Trials.* Oxford: Arnold.

Moore RA; Gavaghan D; Tramer MR; Collins SL; McQway HJ (1998). Size is everything—large amounts of information are needed to overcome random effects in estimating direction and magnitude of treatment effects. *Pain* 78:209–216.

Moseley JB; O'Malley K; Petersen NJ; Menke TJ; Brody BA; Kuykendall DH; Hollingsworth JC; Ashton CM; Wray NP. (2002) A controlled trial of arthroscopic surgery for osteoarthritis of the knee. *N Engl J Med* 347:81–88.

Moye LA. (1998) P-value interpretation and alpha allocation in clinical trials. *Ann Epidemiol* 8:351–357.

Moye LA. (2000) *Statistical Reasoning in Medicine: The Intuitive P-Value Primer.* New York: Springer.

Piantadosi S. (1997) *Clinical Trials: A Methodologic Perspective.* New York: Wiley.

Sacks H; Chalmers TC; Smith H. (1982). Randomized versus historical controls for clinical trials. *Am J Med* 72:233–240.

Schulz KF. (1995). Subverting randomization in controlled trials. *JAMA* 274:1456–1458.

Shuster JJ. (1993). *Practical Handbook of Sample Size Guidelines for Clinical Trials.* Boca Raton, FL: CRC.

Simon R. (1982). Randomized clinical trials and research strategy. *Cancer Treatment Rep* 66:1083–1087.

Simon R. (1999). Bayesian design and analysis of active control clinical trials. *Biometrics* 55:484–487.

Thall PF; Cheng SC. (2001). Optimal two-stage designs for clinical trials based on safety and efficacy. *Stat Med* 20:1023–1032.

Therneau TM; Grambsch PM. (2000) *Modeling survival data.* New York: Springer.

Torgerson D; Campbell M. (1997) Unequal randomisation can improve the economic efficiency of clinical trials. *J Health Serv Res Policy* 2:81–85.

Tubridy N; Ader HJ; Barkhof F; Thompson AJ; Miller DH. (1998) Exploratory treatment trials in multiple sclerosis using MRI: sample size calculations for relapsing-remitting and secondary progressive subgroups using placebo controlled parallel groups. *J Neurol Neurosurg Psychiatry*

Vickers A; Cassileth B; Ernst E et al. (1997). How should we research unconventional therapies? *Int J Technol Assess Health Care* 13:111–121.

Yao Q; Wei LJ. (1996) Play the winner for phase II/III clinical trials. *Stat Med* 15:2413–2423; discussion 2455–2458.

Chapter 7
Exception Handling

THIS CHAPTER IS DEVOTED TO PLANNING for the innumerable petty but essential details—missed appointments, patient complaints, and protocol deviations—that are bound to arise in an extensive and lengthy series of clinical trials. We also consider certain more serious matters such as a high frequency of adverse events that may result in early termination of your study.

PATIENT RELATED

Missed Doses
Phone calls to investigators from patients who have missed a scheduled dose are common. A uniform policy on missed doses should be incorporated in both patient and investigator instructions.

Missed Appointments
Missed appointments are commonplace also, with noncompliant patients being particular offenders. Establish a policy of prior notification by the investigator's office (perhaps a card in the mail a week before the visit and a telephone call the day before). Once again, having a sponsor-paid coordinator at each site helps ensure that your policies are adhered to.

Patients, particularly those whose health has improved or who dislike the treatment, cannot be counted on to reschedule on their own. Have site coordinators follow up immediately by telephone should the patient not appear at the scheduled time.

A Manager's Guide to the Design and Conduct of Clinical Trials, by Phillip I. Good
Copyright ©2006 John Wiley & Sons, Inc.

Suppose (and one should always suppose the worst case as it is inevitable) that the patient fails to appear for the one-month follow-up exam, but does appear at some time before the two-month follow-up. If the patient shows up at five weeks, would this be close enough in time to count as the one-month follow-up? If the patient appears for the first time at seven weeks, would you mark the one-month follow-up as missing and record this exam as the two-month follow-up?

How will you treat patients who show up at other intermediate times? You and your design team need to formulate a consistent policy that will be adhered to throughout the study.

Noncompliance

Noncompliance of patients with the treatment regimen has three chief sources:

1. **Ambiguous directions**
2. **Noncooperative or frightened patients**
3. **Unreported use of concurrent medications**

The first two of these can be dealt with by careful attention to detail during the preparation of patient instructions and the training of personnel who will have direct contact with patients. To deal with the last, questions on concurrent medications, both prescribed and self-administered, should be made part of each follow-up examination.

Adverse Reactions

Physicians are acutely aware of the rare but inevitable instances in which a patient has an immediate adverse reaction to treatment or to the collection and diagnostic procedures associated with treatment. Similarly, any surgical intervention may be accompanied by undesirable events not directly related to the procedure under investigation. You will need to list all such possible reactions and prepare written procedures for dealing with them. This list will become part of your written submission to the regulatory agency.

Reporting Adverse Events

You will require a separate form for recording adverse events that occur during the study and for (possible) reporting to the regulatory agency. This form should provide for both anticipated events (nausea, headache) and unanticipated (other), for the trivial (nausea, headache) and the serious.

The form should note whether the event is continuing or preexisting and (in the investigator's opinion) to what degree it might be related to the intervention. Action(s) taken and its outcome should be noted, along with links to any secondary sets of forms that may have been completed.

Investigators should be instructed to complete and transmit adverse event forms to you as soon as they become aware of the event. As always, computer-assisted data entry facilitates both completion and transmission of such forms.

When Do You Crack the Code?

On receipt of an adverse event form, it should be collated with the set of forms that have already been submitted and two questions addressed:

1. **Are most of the events taking place at a specific site or sites?**
2. **Is a particular event or pattern of events occurring with unusual frequency?**

If the majority of adverse events are occurring at a particular site or sites, the response of your CRMs should be appropriate to the several possibilities: If those sites are treating the majority of the patients—a high proportion of adverse events is to be expected and no further action is required. If those sites are the most conscientious in recording adverse events, the importance of tracking adverse event needs to be stressed with the site coordinators at the remaining sites. If these latter sites may be deviating from the protocol—a visit is warranted.

How you react to an unusually high frequency of adverse events will depend on the severity of the events and whether they were expected or unexpected. An external review panel whose primary concern is the safety of the treatment should review the data concerning the events. The members of this panel should not be regular employees of your company; their skills should mirror those of the members of your design team. Upon this panel's recommendation, the code may be broken and the data in hand subjected to a comprehensive statistical analysis.

Chapter 14 contains a further discussion of this important issue.

INVESTIGATOR RELATED

Lagging Recruitment

Enrollment should be monitored on a continuous basis. Fortunately there is a great deal of commercially available software to help you in this task (see Appendix). Forecasting methods are described in Chapter 14.

Eligibility forms should be completed and transmitted to you on the same day the patient is examined. If only a few sites have lagging enrollments, you are free to concentrate your efforts on those sites. If recruitment is an across-the-board problem, you have five alternatives:

1. Increase the time allotted to complete the trials.
2. Launch an intensive recruiting campaign (see Chapter 9).
3. Recruit additional study centers.
4. Modify the eligibility requirements.
5. Abandon the trials.

Prepare for the worst and have a backup plan ready.

Protocol Deviations

Potential protocol deviations include all of the following:

- **Enrolling ineligible patients**
- **Failing to ensure that each patient has made informed consent**
- **Initiating an intervention other than the one assigned**
- **Altering the nature of the intervention without permission or notification to you**
- **Failing to record data in the manner specified or at the specified times**
- **Recording fraudulent data**

Preventive measures include:

- **Monitoring enrollment procedures**
- **Keeping the intervention and the measurements to be made straightforward and easy to follow**
- **Preparing a detailed, yet easy-to-follow procedures manual (see Chapter 8)**
- **Providing a comprehensive training program (see Chapter 10)**
- **Monitoring the data as they are collected (see Chapters 12 and 13)**

Site-Specific Problems

When lagging enrollments, ineligible patients, patient dropouts, delays in transmittal of forms, protocol deviations, excessive numbers of adverse events, or evidence of fraud can be traced to a few specific sites, then the first obvious step is a visit to the site by the clinical research monitor. In most instances, problems can be resolved through such visits. Perhaps additional training is required, including a detailed walk through the various intervention and recording procedures. Perhaps a visit by the chief investigator to the offending physician(s) may be warranted.

Should such friendly persuasion prove unavailing, you will need to have a plan in place. For minor offenses—too many ineligible patients, too many dropouts, delays in submitting forms—the solution is to do what you would do with any recalcitrant but momentarily essential employee—discontinue further enrollment at the site, spend whatever additional time is necessary to ensure compliance with those patients that are already enrolled, and, above all, pay only for correctly completed forms.

With more serious offenses, your choices are more limited. You will need to notify the regulatory agency of any deviations. The regulatory agency will require that you continue to provide treatment for and monitor the progress of those patients that are currently under the offending physician's care. Legal as well as ethical issues are involved. You don't want to be there.

Preventive measures are essential and include all of the following:

- **Care in recruitment of study physicians and laboratories (see Chapter 9)**
- **Drafting contracts with study physicians and laboratories that spell out the procedural requirements and the penalties for violating them**
- **Monitoring the data as they are collected and taking the earliest possible remedial action.**

Closure

In Chapter 6, we discussed the possibility of an unplanned closure dictated by a high frequency of adverse events. Seldom does an interim analysis reveal a clear-cut pattern: treatment bad, control good or vice versa. More often, the results suggest that external factors are responsible for adverse events or that the events are affecting only a single subgroup such as those with specific risk factors or the most preexisting complications. In such an instance, you may wish to stop enrolling any further members of that subgroup in the study. Only in the event that a single treatment arm appears to be deleterious for all subgroups should the intervention be discontinued and the patients assigned to another treatment arm.

Note: If you discontinue treatment to all patients, you are obligated to notify the regulatory agency and to continue to monitor trial subjects until the scheduled time for termination is reached. Further discussion is in Chapter 14.

Intent to Treat

When an intent-to-treat regimen is adopted, the physician is free to modify or withdraw treatment if warranted by the patient's condition. To turn theory into practice, guidelines for modifications should be established in advance of the trials. Is the physician free to alter the dosage? Or to add an adjunctive therapy? Is she restricted to switching among the protocol alternatives, or may she switch to any treatment she deems appropriate? Have your answers ready before the trials begin.

IS YOUR PLANNING COMPLETE?

Determined the following:

- **Study objectives**
- **Primary responses (efficacy)**
- **Secondary responses (safety)**
- **How responses will be interpreted**
- **Baseline variables**
- **Study population**
- **Time line**
- **Closure**
- **Who will do the monitoring?**

Grouped observations by the individual (or laboratory) making the observations and the time of collection.

Began recruiting for implementation team and study review panels
Completed the trial design:

> **Controls**
> **Randomization**
> **Blinding**
> **Intent to treat**
> **Criteria for acceptance and rejection**
> **Sample size**

Provided for exceptions. You know who will monitor, who will respond to, and how you will deal with the following:

> **Patient-related exceptions**
> **Investigator-related exceptions**
> **Adverse events**
> **Protocol violations**

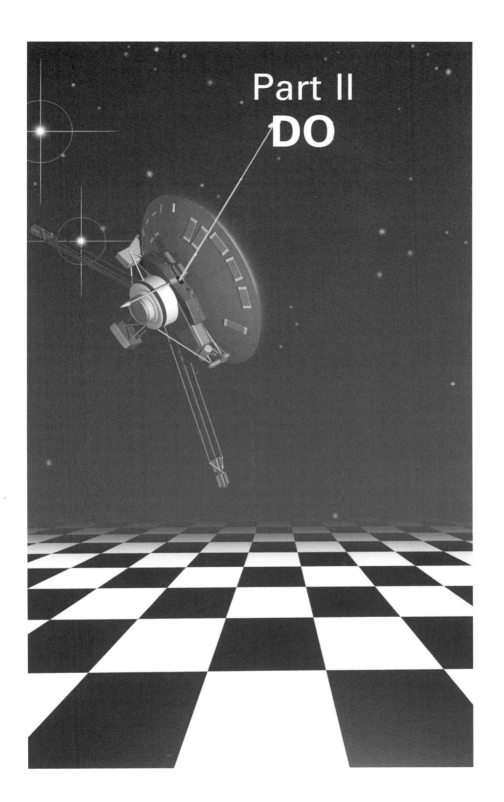

Chapter 8
Documentation

THE PURPOSE OF THIS CHAPTER IS TO DESCRIBE the documentation you must make for the regulatory agency and should make for yourself and your coworkers.

To go ahead with the trials you will need to submit a *proposal* to the regulatory agency.

If you have followed our prescription so far, your design committee will already have prepared a *protocol*, and you will be in the process of designing *procedures manuals* for your investigators and the templates for a series of *interim reports* for use by your staff when monitoring the trials.

Once the trials are complete, you will need to submit one or more final reports to the regulatory agency. You also will need to submit one or more interim reports to them if you are compelled by circumstance to alter the nature of the trials or to terminate the trials before completion. We strongly urge you to utlize the Common Technical Document in making these reports. In fact, since July 2003, use of the common technical document or CTD has been mandatory in Europe and Japan and "highly recommended" by the FDA and Health Canada.

Marketing may ask that you seek to publish your findings. An *AAR* (after action review), discussed in Chapter 16, is the essence of good management.

We cover the scope and contents of all these reports in what follows.

A Manager's Guide to the Design and Conduct of Clinical Trials, by Phillip I. Good
Copyright ©2006 John Wiley & Sons, Inc.

GUIDELINES

Two fundamental rules govern all your written communications with individuals outside your company:

1. **If you and the members of your staff can't follow a report, neither will outside reviewers; the result of sending out such a report will be both potential miscommunication and substantial delays.**
2. **Your submission is a contract; do not commit to tasks you cannot honor or state facts you cannot support.**

COMMON TECHNICAL DOCUMENT

On July 1, 2003, use of the Common Technical Document became mandatory in Europe and Japan and "highly recommended" by the FDA and Health Canada.

The Common Technical Document, or CTD provides an interface for the industry-to-agency transfer of regulatory information. If it functions as intended, it will facilitate the creation, review, life cycle management, and archiving of clinical trial data.

A radical departure from existing documentation is not required; in most instances, the biologic license application or new drug application can be used as a basis for the CTD (Foote, 2004).

CTD specifications provide for printed or electronic submissions, for the format and organization of reports, for the format and contents of tables, and for the format and naming of files and directories.

The CTD provides for analysis of trial data, descriptions of manufacturing processes, and marketing authorization. See, for example, *http://pharmacos.eudra.org/F2/eudralex/vol-2/B/PartIA_032003.doc*.

The CTD does not provide for regional administrative information and prescribing information, amendments, or variations to the initial application. Although CTD specifies page size and type font, each region may also impose its own guidelines—language, for example. In deciding whether one or more of your documents or files are appropriate for use in CTD format, realize that once a particular approach has been adopted, the same approach must be used throughout the life of the dossier.

The CTD is organized into five modules as shown in Figure 8.1. Module 1 is region specific. Modules 2, 3, 4, and 5 are intended to be common for all regions.

Overall organization of the CTD must adhere to the guidelines and may not be modified. Formats of the Nonclinical and Clinical Summaries can be modified to provide the best possible presentation of the technical information.

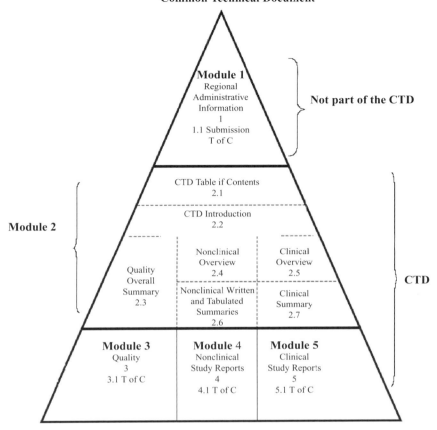

FIGURE 8.1

Module 2 should begin with a general introduction to the pharmaceutical, including its pharmacologic class, mode of action, and proposed clinical use. It should contain seven sections in the following order :

- **CTD Table of Contents**
- **CTD Introduction**
- **Quality Overall Summary**
- **Nonclinical Overview**
- **Clinical Overview**
- **Nonclinical Written and Tabulated Summaries**
- **Clinical Summary**

Documentation is provided for each module on a section-by-section basis at both the FDA website, *http://www.fda.gov/cder/regulatory/ersr/ectd.htm* and the ICH website, *http://www.ich.org/UrlGrpServer.jser?@_ID=276&&_TEMPLATE=254*. CTD guidelines are quite detailed as the following extract from the guidelines for efficacy Module 2, section 2.5: Clinical Overview suggests:

> The Clinical Overview should generally be a relatively short document (about 30 pages) with cross-referencing to more detailed presentations in the Clinical Summary or Module 5 encouraged. The use of graphs and concise tables in the body of the text is encouraged.
>
> The Clinical Overview should present the strengths and limitations of the development program and study results, analyse the benefits and risks of the medicinal product in its intended use, and describe how the study results support critical parts of the prescribing information. In order to achieve these objectives the Clinical Overview should:
>
> - Describe and explain the overall approach to the clinical development of a medicinal product, including critical study design decisions.
> - Assess the quality of the design and performance of the studies, and include a statement regarding GCP compliance.
> - Provide a brief overview of the clinical findings, including important limitations (e.g., lack of comparisons with an especially relevant active comparator, or absence of information on some patient populations, on pertinent endpoints, or on use in combination therapy).
> - Provide an evaluation of benefits and risks based upon the conclusions of the relevant clinical studies, including interpretation of how the efficacy and safety findings support the proposed dose and target indication and an evaluation of how prescribing information and other approaches will optimise benefits and manage risks.
> - Address particular efficacy or safety issues encountered in development, and how they have been evaluated and resolved.
> - Explore unresolved issues, explain why they should not be considered as barriers to approval, and describe plans to resolve them.
> - Explain the basis for important or unusual aspects of the prescribing information.

REPORTING ADVERSE EVENTS

The new *ICH Medical Dictionary for Regulatory Activities* (MedDRA) terminology should be employed in the design of case report forms.

Use MedDRA

- To aggregate reported terms in medically meaningful groupings for the purpose of reviewing and/or analyzing safety data
- To facilitate identification of common data sets for evaluation of clinical and safety information
- To facilitate consistent retrieval of specific cases or medical conditions from a database
- To improve consistency in comparing and understanding "safety signals" and aggregated clinical data
- To facilitate electronic data interchange of clinical safety information
- To report adverse reaction/adverse event (ADR/AE)2 terms via individual case safety reports
- To include ADR/AEs in tables, analyses, and line listings for reports
- To identify frequency of medically similar ADR/AEs
- To capture and present product indications, investigations, medical history, and social history data.

INITIAL SUBMISSION TO THE REGULATORY AGENCY

Not surprisingly, the form of the protocol or investigational plan to be submitted to the regulatory agency closely mirrors the design elements discussed in Chapters 5 and 6. Most of the headings on the accompanying model table of contents should be familiar to you. (The order, content, and titles used in this sample table may need to be varied depending on the requirements of the regulatory agency.)

STUDY PROTOCOL TABLE OF CONTENTS	
Sponsor Data	Early Withdrawal
Introduction: Background and Rationale	Statistical Methods
Objectives	Investigator Responsibilities
Patient Selection	Ethical and Regulatory Considerations
Treatment Plan	Study Committees
Outcome Measures and Evaluation	Appendices
Procedures	Bibliography
Clinical Follow-Up	Sample informed consent form
Adverse Events	Schedule of events
Data Management, Monitoring, Quality Control	

Sponsor Data

Sponsor data should include the name, address, and telephone number of your company, the name and title of the chief investigator, and the name, title, phone number, and e-mail address of your regulatory agency liaison.

Justifying the Study

Your justification should be that originally presented to the executive committee. Begin by stating the prevalence of the disease condition you propose to treat, along with its effects. Here is an example: "Colorectal cancer is the second most common visceral malignancy in the United States. An estimated 156,000 new cases of the disease will occur. . . ."

The balance of your justification should briefly summarize previous work you and other investigators have done that would lead one to believe that the intervention you propose will be both safe and efficacious. Include data from any or all of the following sources:

- **Pharmacology and biochemical theory—describe the mechanism of action if known**
- **Animal experiments—include toxicology findings**
- **Anecdotal studies**
- **Case-control studies**
- **Short-term clinical studies including Phase I determinations of the maximum tolerated dose and Phase II studies of the minimum effective dose.**

You should also reference any previous full-scale clinical studies when you are proposing extensions of the subject population, modifications to the treatment regimen, or new indications for use of an already-marketed intervention.

Brief descriptions of each study should be provided, along with journal and text references where available.

Again, note that what distinguishes the full-scale clinical study (termed Phase III in the United States) from prior clinical trials is that it entails measures of both safety and efficacy, involves a predetermined dose or treatment regimen, is long term (at least a year in length), and includes sufficiently many patients that accurate estimates of the incidence of all but the rarest of side effects can be made.

Take pains to differentiate your proposal from prior work. For example, "The proposed study will include both men and women. It will involve more than 10 times the number of patients observed in any single previous study. The study period of one year is eight months in excess of any previous study period."

Remember, the object of your proposal is to convince even the most conservative and cautious reader that the investigation you propose is both prudent (because it is solidly grounded in prior efforts) and desirable (because the study's depth and breadth ensure that the public will be fully protected once the study is complete).

Objectives

This section as well as each of the remaining sections of your proposal should be largely self-standing. Although this will lead to substantial redundancy, it facilitates the review process and forestalls misunderstandings.

This section should begin with a focused restatement of what you outlined in your introduction and include brief definitions of the primary and secondary end points.

Patient Selection

Provide comprehensive listings of the inclusion and exclusion criteria you will employ. (Reminder: any limitations will also limit the scope of subsequent marketing of the intervention.)

Here is an example:

"Eligibility Criteria

To be eligible for this study a patient must satisfy the following criteria:

- **Be between 30 and 80 years of age.**
- **Have a physician's assessment of good general health with an expected survival of at least five years.**
- **Have the ability and willingness to understand informed consent and to comply with study procedures.**
- **Not currently undergoing treatment in a chemoprevention trial.**
- **Not pregnant or nursing. Women of childbearing potential must be willing to use an effective method of birth control throughout the study.**
- **Have histologically proven colon or rectal cancer."**

"Exclusion Criteria

To be eligible for this study a patient may not have any of the following diagnosed health conditions:

- **More than 100 polyps at the time of resection**
- **Active invasive malignancy, other than nonmelanoma skin cancer.**

- Cardiovascular disease, NYHA Class 3 or 4.
- Immunosuppressive therapy within the six months preceding the intake appointment. Nonimmunosuppressive therapy steroid therapy does NOT necessitate exclusion from the study.
- Clinically obvious narcotic and/or alcohol dependence within the six months preceding the intake appointment.
- History of ulcerative colitis or Crohn disease."

Treatment Plan

This section should include the following:

- Time line for the trials
- Brief description of the experimental design, including the extent of the blinding and the method(s) to be employed to ensure the blinding is sustained throughout the course of the trials
- Sample size
- Method of treatment assignment
- Rules governing early termination or modification of the protocol

Outcome Measures and Evaluation

This section incorporates a more detailed and precise discussion of the end points listed under the heading of objectives. Describe how and by whom each measurement will be taken and how and by whom each measurement will be evaluated.

Procedures

This section includes brief descriptions of any invasive procedures as well as of specimen collection and handling. It should also include methods for handling any possible adverse reactions to procedures. For studies involving medications, the following must be included:

- Dosage form (capsule, tablet, ointment)
- Route of administration (oral, intramuscular, intravenous)
- Frequency of administration

For intravenous administration include the rate of administration and the concentration of the medication in the delivery medium.

Clinical Follow-Up

Provide tabular summaries of any required testing and any other follow-up procedures as in Table 8.1. In other words, expand on the time line covered under the treatment plan. Also, you will need to describe:

- Any concomitant medical therapy

TABLE 8.1 Schedule of Events

	Screen	Surgery	Two weeks	One month	Six months	Eight months	One year
History	√						
Consent	√						
ECG	√	√			√		
WBC	√	√	√	√			
creatinine	√	√					
cholesterol	√						
CK&CKMB	√	√					
ACT		√					
Follow-up			phone	√	√		√
Angiogram	√	√				√	

- Procedures for dealing with withdrawals and noncompliant patients
- Extent of any further follow-up examinations after the termination of the study

Adverse Events

List the most likely adverse events, along with how you plan to monitor and report on them. Here is an example from a study of the effects of aspirin.

> A questionnaire will be completed for each patient at each follow-up visit. The questionnaire specifically addresses gastrointestinal symptoms (nausea, vomiting, heartburn, dyspepsia), abdominal pain, and bleeding.
>
> Patients will also be encouraged to report any side effects as they occur and will be provided with an information sheet containing the local coordinator's telephone number.
>
> A physical examination will be conducted at each follow-up visit and any new medical conditions will be recorded. Laboratory tests will be performed as the physician determines.

Data Management, Monitoring, Quality Control

Briefly describe the use of computer-aided data entry. State that all data entry screens will be incorporated as part of the final submission. (See under e-Subs later in this chapter.)

Statistical Analysis

Describe the analytical measurement(s) to be made, the relevance to the protocol objectives, and the statistical methodology to be utilized. Be brief—a textbook is not required. Specify the analytical plan to be

> **FILL IN THE HOLES**
>
> Your protocol should not only describe *how* the data are to be analyzed but *which* data are to be used for the analysis. Take into account *all* contingencies. Here's an example from an (almost) successful study.
>
> "The appropriate angiogram to use for follow-up purposes is to be determined as follows:
>
> 1. If a patient had a target site revascularization after 14 days and prior to 7.5 months, the angiogram immediately preceding the surgery will be used. If not, then
> 2. The first follow-up angiogram within 8 ± 0.5 months after the index procedure will be used. If such an angiogram is not available, then
> 3. Use a follow-up angiogram performed at least 4 months after the index intervention. Otherwise,
> 4. If there is objective evidence of recurrent ischemia between 14 days and 4 months and repeat angiography during the same period demonstrates restenosis, that angiogram will be analyzed as the follow-up angiogram. If such angiograms are not available, then
> 5. An angiogram taken within 12 months will be used."

used for the protocol measurement(s). Include the criteria and procedures used to assess analytical results. Cite all relevant scientific literature supporting the use of the analytical method for the intended measurements.

Here is an example: "The difference in recurrence rates between the aspirin and the placebo groups will be tested with Fisher's exact test. A preliminary exact test will be performed to see if the data from all cites may be combined. (See Good, 2005, page 117–8.) Sample size was chosen so as to have 90% power to detect a 10% difference in recurrence rates with a test at the 5% significance level."[24]

Investigator Responsibilities

This section should include explicit statements to the effect that the investigator will not

- **utilize the experimental intervention outside the scope of the study;**
- **undertake investigative procedures on any enrolled patient other than those specified in the protocol; or**
- **publish the results of their experience with the intervention until the publication of the multicenter results**

---

[24]The statistical terms were defined in Chapter 6.

and will

- administer and obtain informed consent from all patients;
- administer the intervention and record and report measurements only as specified in the protocol;
- submit all data and supporting documents in a timely fashion;
- return any unused drugs or devices at the conclusion of the study; and
- retain copies of all patient records as specified by regulatory agency (and your own) requirements.

This section should also be incorporated in the procedures manual you give to each physician.

Ethical and Regulatory Considerations

This section is required by some but not all regulatory agencies, and its form and content will depend on which branch of the regulatory agency is responsible for supervising your trials. Analogous to the preceding section, it consists of a listing of your company's responsibilities with respect to the patients, the investigators, and the regulatory agency. It is a form of contract (as is the entire submission), and you as the manager are responsible for seeing that its pledges are honored.

Study Committees

Possible study committees include an executive board (consisting of you, your regulatory affairs liaison, and the chief investigators), a

---

IF YOU DON'T HAVE ANYTHING TO SAY . . .

The protocol is not a term paper; your objective is not merely to cover a piece of paper with words, but to provide a detailed description of what you propose to do. KISS.

Consider the following example of what *not* to write taken in its entirety from an actual Bumbling proposal:

"Secondary Response Variables and Multivariable Modeling

Many secondary response variables may be evaluated. The measurable responses fall under two broad testing categories:

1. Subgroup hypotheses that utilize the primary hypothesis end points for potentially important patient strata, e.g., long stents, use without extended surgery, restenosis in women, diabetics, or the left descending artery

2. Secondary hypotheses that require separate end points for analysis (e.g., costs or vascular complications). The secondary questions will be confined to three categories: i) other definitions of restenosis, ii) complications, iii) other."

safety board (consisting of at least two physicians and a biostatician who are not directly involved in the conduct of the trials), a clinical events adjudication committee (consisting of at least three physicians who are specialists in the medical area and are not directly involved in the conduct of the trials), and other review panels specific to the investigation (e.g., pathology review, angiogram review).

Appendixes

In addition to a list of the journals and books that were cited in your proposal and a sample informed consent form, any or all of the following may be required depending on the requirements of your regulatory agency:

1. **List of investigators accompanied by copies of instructions provided to them**
2. **List of laboratories participating in the study accompanied by copies of instructions provided to them**
3. **List of personnel with access to treatment codes**

Before making any submission, be sure to consult the new drug/device application of the appropriate agency. In the United States, consult *http://www.fda.gov/opacom/morechoices/industry/guidedc.htm*.

SAMPLE INFORMED CONSENT FORM

Introduction

Purpose of the Study

Randomization Procedure

- If you agree to participate in this study, you will randomly (by chance) be assigned to either [describe treatment] or [describe alternative(s)]. You have a 50-50 chance to receive either treatment. Your physician will decide before randomization whether the addition of [a proposed adjunctive therapy] is necessary.

Procedure

[Include only a brief description adopting the patient's point of view.]

Potential Risks

- The risks of this intervention [name] are very similar to [name the alternative intervention and describe the risks associated with it].

- (if warranted) As with any measurements of this type, there are certain risks, which include dye or drug allergy, and . . .
- (if applicable) The use of [name the adjunct therapy] is standard in all treatments of your condition and entails the following risks: [list].

Potential Benefits

- Studies such as this are performed to determine the relative risk and benefits of these treatments. No definite benefits can be guaranteed by your participation in this study.

Confidentiality

[Assure the patient that his/her identity is protected.]

Alternative Courses of Treatment

- The following . . . and . . . are accepted standard treatments for your disease condition. If after consideration of these potential benefits and risks you do not wish to participate in the study, you and your doctor will decide which standard treatment may be appropriate for you.

Policy Regarding Research Related Injuries

- In the event of injury resulting from your participation in this study there will be no monetary compensation or subsidized medical treatment provided to you by any person involved in this research project including the study sponsor or [name of the institution].

Payments or Additional Costs to Patients

- There are no payments to patients participating in this study. The routine cost for this procedure will be billed to your insurance carrier. Nonroutine costs required by this study protocol [name them] will be paid by the sponsor.

Problems or Questions

Patient's Consent

I have read the explanation about this study and have been given the opportunity to discuss it and to ask questions. I hereby consent to take part in this study.

Signature of Participant	Date
Signature of Investigator	Date
Signature of Witness	Date

PROCEDURES MANUALS

The design process is not complete until you have prepared a detailed list of the information that is to be gathered (see Chapter 9) and a manual of the procedures that are to be followed in gathering and evaluating the information.

We've already noted the variation that is inherent when we move from one patient to the next. With some interventions, there can be just as much variation in *how* the treatment is administered. With all interventions, there can be considerable variation in how the observations are made, even those on a single patient, unless we are consistent in the manner in which we measure them. Moreover, if measurements are made on two different patients by two different investigators, then added to the normal patient-to-patient variation would be differences that result from differences in technique. The object of your procedures manual is to minimize these differences.

The manual should be the joint product of study physicians and professional writers. A separate manual should be prepared for each investigational laboratory and review panel.

Physician's Procedures Manual

After a brief reiteration of the purpose of the trials, the physician's manual should contain the following detailed instructions:

- **Determining eligibility.** Define each criterion, explain its purpose, and note the requirement for strict adherence. Give step-by-step instructions for obtaining the necessary information. (For example, the eligibility questionnaire is to be completed by the patient initially and then is to be gone over item by item with the patient by the physician or the study nurse.)
- **Making and recording each of the necessary baseline and follow-up measurements.** Note who is to take the observations (nurse, nurse practitioner, only the physician) and how measurements are to be recorded (include units). If materials are to be sent to an outside laboratory, describe how samples are to be collected and provide packing and shipping instructions.
- **Administering the intervention.** Preface by noting the following restrictions:
    - Experimental intervention can only be used with enrolled patients.
    - Intervention cannot begin until eligibility and specified baseline data have been submitted and an assignment made to treatment.
    - Intervention cannot be stopped or modified without first notifying you, the sponsor of the trials.
    - The only investigative procedures that may be used on an enrolled patient are those specified in the protocol.

    Provide a step-by-step description of the procedure. If surgery is involved, the text should be accompanied by pictures and,

> preferably, by a videotape, compact disk, or DVD illustrating the procedure.
- **Reporting of adverse events.** What events are likely; how they will be detected; how they will be summarized; how they will be reported.

Include a section on patient compliance. Here is a possible wording: "Every patient contact should be used to educate, motivate, and reinforce compliance. Individualized caring attention by the members of your staff will also increase patient adherence to the prescribed therapy."

Incorporate any sample instructions you want the physician to pass on to the patient. For example, "One pill is to be taken twice a day with meals. In the event that you forget to take a pill at the designated time, please take it as soon as possible. If you miss a dose completely, please do not double up on the dose, but simply take your pill at the next regularly scheduled time. I'd also like you to make a record of any doses you do miss and to give me the list the next time you are in the office."

These instructions should be included as an appendix to the physician procedures manual in a form that lends itself to copying and distribution to patients.

Laboratory Guidelines

The laboratory guidelines prepared for each individual specialty laboratory should be as comprehensive as those provided to the physician. They should cover the preparation of the sample, shipping and receiving, and the particulars of the analysis and should be as detailed as possible.

This latter section should be written only after receiving a preliminary description from the laboratory. Although it may seem foolish to create a document that merely parrots back the laboratory's own words, the result is to create a contract and, hopefully, to ensure uniformity in technique throughout the length of the trials.

INTERIM REPORTS

Your interim reports consist of all reports that are essential to successful conduct of the study. Included are reports on enrollment, submission of scheduled follow-up data, adverse events, and an ongoing abstract of findings.

TABLE 8.2 Interim Enrollment Report (1/6/03–1/7/03)

Site	Patients Enrolled	Enrollment Target	Prospect Interviews	Women Enrolled	Minority Enroll	Comments
002	8	17	11	2	0	
003	11	13	20	0	0	Must enroll women.
004	0	6	0	0	0	Drop? Did not return call.
005	5	20	10	0	5	TV ads begin Monday.
006	10	15	15	2	3	
007	8	13	8	?	?	Some forms not entered.
...	...	...	...	...	...	...
018	50	66	85	9	5	

TABLE 8.3 Angiogram Status and Follow-up Rate Tracking (3/3/04)

Site	Patients Enrolled	Follow-Up Angio Not Done	Follow-Up Missing	Patients for Analysis	Follow-Up Rate*	Comments
002	17	0		17	100%	
003	13	5	2	6	46%	Core lab has all films.
004	6	3		3	50%	
005	20	5		15	75%	
006	15	4		11	73%	
...						
018	66	20	5	41	62%	Core lab has 1; site is locating 3 others; 1 is unavailable.

Enrollment Report

"As of 1 May 2003, 221 (52%) of the 400 anticipated patients are enrolled. This number includes 128 Caucasian, 26 African-American, 14 Hispanic, and 24 subjects designating themselves as Asian or other. A total of 856 potential subjects were interviewed. Sites 2, 4, and 8 have recruited 100%, 95%, and 80% of their expectations. Sites 5, 6, and 9 have not yet recruited any patients."

In the hypothetical case depicted in Table 8.2, enrollment has passed the halfway mark, yet one of the sites has not recruited a single patient. What are you going to do about it?

Data in Hand

"As of 1 August 2003, 338 initial follow-up reports from the 385 enrolled patients are in hand. 20 reports are overdue, including 5 from site 10. Laboratory results from 28 of these patients are missing or incomplete (see Table 8.3). 145 patients report partial or complete improvement on the self-diagnostic scale. 40 patients report worsening symptoms. "

TABLE 8.4a Adverse Events by Treatment

Date of First Intervention 1 Aug 2003	Current Date: 26 Sept. 2003	
	With ABC	Without
Q-wave MI	2	1
Non-Q-wave MI	5	10
Angina	1	1
Chest pains	8	4
Bleeding complications	4	1
...		
Other	3	5

TABLE 8.4b Adverse Events/Patient

# Adv Events	With ABC	Without	Total
0	233	253	486
1	56	46	102
2	30	33	63
3	21	17	38
4	16	13	29
...	...	...	...
11	1	0	1
Total	300	294	594

TABLE 8.4c Adverse Events by Period

Period	With ABC	Without	Total
Procedure	45	30	75
Two weeks	8	6	14
One month	39	24	63
...			
Six months	32	26	58
...	...	...	...
Total	300	294	594

Adverse Event Report

Three types of interim adverse event reports are of interest: 1) frequency of specific adverse events by treatment, 2) number of adverse events per patient by treatment, and 3) adverse events by time period and treatment. The form of these reports is illustrated in Tables 8.4a,b,c.

ANNOTATED ABSTRACT

An HTML format provides links to lists of missing data, protocol logic, and analysis software.

Prepared by Phillip Good July 30, 2001 using 12 July 2001 database
Company Confidential. For internal use only.
Among 705 patients, 28% of the 702 patients for whom data was available were females, and the mean age for the 702 patients for whom birth data was available was 63.9 ± 4.6.
- *Click here to see a list of patients with missing or erroneous dates.*
- *Click here to view program logic*
- *Click here to view SAS programs*

The 658 angiographic films analyzed showed average lesion length to be 12.5 ± 1.9 mm.
- *Click here to see a list of patients with missing film data.*
- *Click here to view program logic*
- *Click here to view SAS programs*

RVD was 2.76 ± 0.51 mm (n = 624).
- *Click here to see lists of patients with missing measurements.*
- *Click here to view program logic*
- *Click here to view SAS program*

Complex lesions were identified as long (≥12 mm but ≤32 mm) 54%, extra long (>32 mm) 4.3%, ostial 5%, and bifurcation 28% based on the results of 700 patients. Complex lesions were identified as CTO 4% based on the results of 699 patients.
- *Click here to see a list of patients whose eligibility forms are not on file.*
- *Click here to view program logic*
- *Click here to view SAS program*

Thirty-day MACE included 1 death, 3 Q-wave MI, and 10 non-Q-wave MI.
- *Click here to see a list of patients with missing film data.*
- *Click here to view program logic*
- *Click here to view SAS programs*

Postprocedural residual stenosis based on reports from 670 patients was 17.0% ± 2.1% in the traditional device group and 13.0% ± 1.4% in the novel device group.
- *Click here to see a list of patients with missing treatment assignments.*
- *Click here to view program logic*
- *Click here to view SAS programs*

Binary residual stenosis based on an analysis of angiograms of the target lesion from 450 patients was 21.9% in the traditional group and 18.2% in the novel group.
- *Click here to see a list of patients with missing data.*
- *Click here to view program logic*
- *Click here to view SAS programs*

Program Logic

Age
Age is determined for each patient by matching the procedure starting date with the birth date.

Lesion length
Average lesion length is calculated by taking the mean of the pre-procedural lesion lengths.

RVD
RVD is computed as the average of the actual, not the interpolated, preprocedural measurements.

Complex Lesions
The source of the information was the [prm] database.
Patients with no eligibility form on file were eliminated.
Records for events other than preprocedural or procedural were eliminated. If both records were present for the same patient, only the latter was used. Duplicate records were eliminated.

A lesion was
- long if $12 \leq LGTH \geq 32$; xtralong if $LGTH > 32$;
- ostial if segloc = 04
- bifurcation if lsnbch = 02 or bifurc = 04
- CTO IF event_id = "PROC" AND pag_name = "11_INITL" AND lsnocl = 02 or 03.

MACE
Deaths derived from outcome database with otcm = = 63.
Number of Q-wave MI and non Q-wave MI derived from outcome database with cls = = 9003 or 9004.
Time after procedure of adverse event was determined by subtracting the procedure starting date from the date of the event.

> PRS
> Postprocedure residual stenosis (PRS) is calculated from the postprocedure lesion MLD (the average of two measurements) and the postprocedure RVD.
>
> BR
> For those patients who had follow-up angiograms, binary restenosis (BR) is defined as restenosis $\geq 50\%$ where restenosis is calculated from the follow-up target lesion MLD (the average of two measurements) and the RVD.
>
> If angiography demonstrated binary restenosis at the target lesion between 14 days and 7 months and 2 weeks the patient was counted as having BR. Otherwise, a follow-up angiogram of the target lesion at 8 ± 0.5 months was used. If such an angiogram was not available, the first angiogram of the target lesion taken after 4 months was used as the basis of determination.

FINAL REPORT(S)

Although it may seem curious that we would discuss the final report before we've even begun to collect data, the form of the final report(s) should be envisioned during the design process and only the numbers remain to be filled in during the analysis phase. It is our reports that should determine the nature of the data we collect. By preparing the form of the final report now, we have the opportunity to uncover any remaining discrepancies.

The necessary reports include ongoing summaries (interim and final), a comprehensive report for the regulatory agency, and journal articles.

Regulatory Agency Submissions

The final report to the regulatory agency, like the interim abstract, should appear (and be) concise while providing links to detailed expositions. These latter should provide further links to summary tables and figures and, eventually, to the raw data itself. ICH (1996) should be consulted for overall guidelines.

Prefatory material should identify your project with its name, an alphanumerical ID if one was supplied by the regulatory agency, and your sponsor data so that the report can be immediately linked to the proposal that you submitted originally. Next should come a single summary paragraph outlining the form of the study and stating the principal results. Here is an example:

> **400 patients with a prior history of... received a control treatment of ... in a single-blind intent-to-treat study, while 385 patients received a ... plus.... The binary restenosis rate of 23.2% for the control patients was significantly greater than the rate of 18.2% for the group receiving... plus.... The control group experienced more deaths and a statistically greater number of non-Q wave MI's than those receiving the new treatment.**

Further paragraphs should be used to expound on the following topics:

- **Demographics.** For example, "the experience of the males and females in the group were similar (see Table 1); those with fewer initial complications benefited the most from the new treatment (see Table 2)."
- **Nature and frequency of adverse events, by type and treatment. Events should be classified by severity and by their relation to the intervention. Note whether a safety committee reviewed the events.**
- **Exceptions. Tabulate withdrawals, noncompliance, and modifications in treatment by starting treatment.**

Reproduce those sections of the protocol (updated to reflect any changes) dealing with end points and your measurement and recording methods.

Tabular material, e.g., Table 1 on the differing experiences of males and females, should be accompanied by a discussion of the statistical techniques employed and include measures of variability (23.2% ± 4.6%), of sample size (n = 323), and of statistical significance (p < 2%). It also should include links to the data extraction and analyses programs so that the results may be independently validated.

Almost all the statistical analyses you perform will require you to first group the data. For example, you will want to combine the data from the various treatment sites, or from all patients regardless of sex or number of risk factors. You will have to precede your analyses by a justification of this grouping, that is, you will have to demonstrate there are no statistically significant differences in result among the categories you wish to group.[25] These preliminary analyses form an essential part of your final report.

---

[25]If significant differences exist among the categories, you will have to present separate tabulations for each distinct group. (For a more extensive discussion of this point, see Chapter 15.)

e-Subs

> A reviewer cannot refuse an electronic submission.—CDER Commitments, 1998

Your final submission to the regulatory agency will be in two parts: a printed copy of your final report and an electronic copy of your database and the programs you're used to retrieve and analyze the data. In the United States, the latter is termed an e-sub or CANDA (Computer-Aided New Drug Application).

CANDAs, and computer-assisted product licensing applications submitted for vaccines and other biological products, shorten review time by reducing the need to sift through reams of paper to get the answers to reviewers' questions. Ordinarily, if a medical reviewer has a question about a specific patient in a drug trial, the reviewer sends a written request for the patient's record to the central document room where new drug application files are kept. It could take a day or more to get the information. Moreover, reviewing scientists often need to go back to you, the drug sponsor, for clarification or reworking of statistical data, which can delay the process for weeks. CANDAs eliminate much of this delay.

By employing computer-assisted data entry you are automatically in a position to submit a CANDA.

Between 1991 and 1994, CANDAs in the United States were approved about 6 months faster than traditional paper applications—in an average of 18.4 months compared with about 24.6 months. The FDA hopes that eventually all new drug applications will contain data that can be processed by computer. See also Agency Perspective on Electronic Submissions (as of 1998) at *http://www.fda.gov/cder/present/disom/index.htm*

Whether or not you submit a CANDA, you will still need to provide the regulatory agency with access to the database if requested and provide the agency with the details of the software used in the analysis.

Journal Articles

Drafting and publishing journal articles provides ammunition for your marketing department. They'll use quotes such as the following in your ads, "As reported in *JAMA* (or *Lancet*, or *Biotechnology Today*), our new product provides relief in 50% more cases." Your field representatives will give out copies of the articles to physicians as part of your product's information packet.

Five rules apply:

1. **Your article should mirror your report to the regulatory agency (though you may omit the material dealing with noncompliant patients and other exceptions).**
2. **Submit your article first to the top, high-circulation journals and work your way down.**
3. **Follow the guidelines for submission each journal provides.**
4. **"Describe statistical methods with enough detail to enable a knowledgeable reader with access to the data to verify the reported results.[26]"**
5. **Utilize CONSORT flow charts and checklists.** *http://www.consort-statement.org/.*

The CONSORT statement is available in several languages and has been endorsed by prominent medical journals such as *The Lancet, Annals of Internal Medicine*, and the *Journal of the American Medical Association*. Its use is the guarantee of integrity in the reported results of research.

CONSORT comprises a checklist and flow diagram to help improve the quality of reports of randomized controlled trials. The checklist includes items, based on evidence, that need to be addressed in the report; the flow diagram provides readers with a clear picture of the progress of all participants in the trial, from the time they are randomized until the end of their involvement. The intent is to make the experimental process more clear, flawed or not, so that users of the data can more appropriately evaluate its validity for their purposes.

Don't trust one of your investigators to prepare the article unless he or she has a track record of successful publication. Normally, your marketing department should be able to provide a professional writer to work with the investigator. If not, hire one.

FOR FURTHER INFORMATION

The Asilomar Working Group on Recommendations for Reporting Clinical Trials in the Biomedical Literature. (1996) Checklist of information for inclusion in reports of clinical trials. *Ann Inter Med* 124:741–743.

Begg C; Cho M; Eastwood S; Horton R; Moher D; Olkin I et al. (1996) Improving the quality of reporting of randomized controlled trials: The CONSORT Statement. *JAMA* 276:637–639.

---

[26]Quote is that of the International Committee of Medical Journal Editors (1991).

Expert Working Group (Efficacy) of the International Conference on Harmonisation of Technical Requirements for Registration of Pharmaceuticals for Human Use (ICH). *Guideline for Industry: Structure and Content of Clinical Reports.* 1996. *http://www.fda.gov/cder/guidance/iche3.pdf Federal Register* (61 FR 37320)

Foote M. (2004) Using the biologic license application or new drug application as a basis for the common technical document. *Biotechnol Annu Rev* 10:251–258.

Good PI. (2005) *Resampling Methods.* Boston: Birkhauser. 3rd Ed.

International Committee of Medical Journal Editors (1991). Uniform requirements for manuscripts submitted to biomedical journals. *N Engl J Med* 324:424–428. (Since replaced by the CONSORT statement.)

Kessler DA. (1997) Remarks by the Commissioner of Food and Drugs. *Food Drug Law J* 52:1–5.

Long TA; Secic M. (1997) *How to Report Statistics in Medicine.* Philadelphia: American College of Physicians.

O'Connor M; Woodford FP. (1976) *Writing Scientific Papers in English.* Amsterdam: Elsevier.

Rutman O; Givens SV. (1997) Evolution of the CANDA at Roche. *J Biopharm Stat* 7:605–615.

Switula D. (2000) Principles of good clinical practice (GCP) in clinical research. *Sci Eng Ethics* 6:71–77.

Chapter 9
Recruiting and Retaining Patients and Physicians

SELECTING YOUR CLINICAL SITES

Two factors should guide you in selecting clinical sites for multicenter trials:

1. **Diversifying the demographics of prospective patient populations**
2. **Avoiding competition in recruiting patients.**

One of the most effective ways to diversify your patient demographics is to make your trials transnational. Different cultures have different eating habits, different customs; their physicians have different prescribing patterns. If your trials are to be limited to a single country, make sure that your trials include patients in both rural and urban areas, private as well as public hospitals.

You don't want to be trying to recruit patients in areas where the more likely prospects are already participating in the clinical trials of your competitors. To avoid problems, consult CenterWatch's Drugs in Clinical Trials Database (*http://www.centerwatch.com/professional/ cwpipeline/*) or that of Current Controlled Trials, *http://www. controlled-trials.com/*. These are comprehensive online resources offering detailed profiles of new investigational treatments in Phase I through III clinical trials. Updated weekly, CenterWatch's online directory provides information on more than 2000 drugs for more than 800 disease conditions worldwide in a well-organized and easy-to-reference format. Detailed profile information is provided for each drug.

A Manager's Guide to the Design and Conduct of Clinical Trials, by Phillip I. Good
Copyright ©2006 John Wiley & Sons, Inc.

These databases are ideal resources for monitoring the performance of drugs in clinical trials; tracking competitors' development activity; identifying development partners; and identifying clinical grant opportunities.

RECRUITING PHYSICIANS

Your overall objective is to recruit physicians who can provide and care for the large number of eligible patients your study requires within the time period you've allotted for the study.

Ideally, all trials would be conducted at a single site. This would keep costs to a minimum, ensure greater control over protocol administration, and eliminate the need for your statistician to correct for site-to-site differences. It's not going to happen. Still, you'll want to keep the number of sites to a minimum. Group practices, clinical research centers, and teaching hospitals are to be preferred to solo practitioners.

Obviously, your first choice for the panel will be physicians you've worked with successfully on other projects. A measure of caution is needed even here. Sometimes such physicians turn into "contract professionals." They spend insufficient time with study patients or, because they are already participating in several other studies, may not have sufficient time to devote to yours. They may no longer be sufficiently stringent with regard to eligibility criteria. Or may they try to shape the results toward what they perceive as your expectations. Even with physicians you know well, a preliminary on-site inspection is essential.

One can also try to recruit friends of "friends," that is, individuals referred by field representatives and existing investigators, but this procedure offers no particular advantages over a straightforward solicitation of all the investigators in a given area. Your focus should not be on friendship but on which physician's practice is likely to yield the most eligible patients.

A clinician on your staff should make initial contact with potential investigators. McBride et al. (1996) report that mailing to individual physicians, a cumbersome and expensive method, has a very low response rate. Initial contacts with practice medical directors increase the participation rate substantially, and recruitment meetings with local practitioners improve both study participation and practice-project communication. Other important factors in recruiting and retaining investigators according to Carey et al. (1996) are close liaison with local medical organizations; ongoing personal contact

> **RECRUIT WITH CARE**
>
> "Thirteen leading medical journals will today warn that the promise of financial rewards is corrupting human clinical trials.
>
> "The editors will criticise pharmaceuticals companies for their use of private nonacademic research groups—called contract research organizations (CROs)—instead of scientists connected to universities and hospitals."
> *Financial Times*, 10 September 2001.
>
> A list of investigators who have repeatedly or deliberately failed to comply with FDA regulatory requirements for studies or have submitted false information to the study's sponsor is found at *http://www.fda.gov/ora/compliance_ref/ bimo/dis_res_assur.htm*

with the practices; and ongoing recognition of the value of the practicing physician's time.

Teaching Hospitals

Your second obvious choice, a teaching hospital staffed by research-oriented physicians who are almost guaranteed to see a large numbers of patients satisfying your inclusion criteria, has at least two major drawbacks:

The first is the patients themselves, a large proportion of whom, being indigent, have had substandard or no medical care in the past and thus present an entire constellation of symptoms and underlying etiologies in addition to those of primary interest.

The second is that academic physicians, professors, and fellows at medical schools and research institutions, while understanding your need for a double-blind approach, thorough documentation, and patient consent forms, generally have experience only with smaller studies of more limited scope. Industry-sponsored trials often entail a 30- to 50-page protocol in contrast to the 5- to 10-page protocols common in the academic area, and industry collection forms can range from 50 to 200 pages per patient, in contrast to the 5- to 10-page forms of the typical academic trial. Academic research is typically completed in months rather than years, with the result that physicians drawn from teaching hospitals may prove less and less cooperative as trials continue, particularly if, in the later stages, it appears there are unlikely to be any publishable results.

Clinical Resource Centers

A third resource is profit-based clinical resource centers that have been set up specifically to conduct clinical trials. An annotated guide to centers in the United States may be found at *http://www.centerwatch.com/*.

A typical listing in this guide might note the number of trials the center has assisted in, the number of resident physicians, their backgrounds and clinical trials experience, and their medical specialties. One center in these listings advertises a single investigator supported by "five highly qualified clinical research coordinators, with an average of five years in pharmaceutical research each; three of the study coordinators are CCRC certified." As an additional bonus, this center provides "a database of over 12,465 clinical research volunteers. In addition, the center has access to a database of more than 35,000 patients from two private practices."

As you did when you hired a contractor to add a room to your house, probe well beyond the advertisement to establish the facts.

Look to Motivations

Let's suppose you have gathered together a group of physicians who you feel are capable of recruiting and working with patients during the time period you have allotted for the study and that you have visited their offices and operating wards and are convinced they would make desirable members of the team. How can you persuade them to come aboard?

Consider the following eleven motivators listed by Spilker (1991):

1. **Enhance one's career (a priority for academic physicians, it can also function as a demotivator if the trial does not appear to be paying off)**
2. **Participate in scientifically exciting research**
3. **Obtain medical benefits for one's patients**
4. **Obtain new medical or scientific equipment provided by sponsors to enable trial (or purchased with monies available downstream)**
5. **Obtain new staff to help with clinical trial (this motivator could backfire as the physician begins to think of the staff as his own and wants to assign them to other tasks)**
6. **Obtain money that may be used for personal interests**
7. **Obtain money that may be used to conduct unsponsored trails of personal and professional interest**
8. **Publish scientifically and medically important journal articles**
9. **Develop a long-term relationship with you and your firm**
10. **Repay a favor (can only be pushed so far)**
11. **Be part of a team (this latter motivator is particularly important for physicians engaged in a solo practice or who, for a variety of reasons, feel estranged from their coworkers)**

Physician Retention

Don't go overboard on the sales pitch. There is no point in recruiting physicians who are not going to remain with the study or, worse, who remain on the payroll but do not contribute.

The first rule in successful retention is not to hire the wrong investigators to begin with. Some physicians may not be good candidates because of too strong a belief in one modality or another. Others may have been guilty of misconduct or of nonadherence to protocol in a prior trial.

No investigator should be brought on board without at least two interviews and a visit (not a telephone call) to the local medical society. Your sales representatives can be particularly helpful in providing feedback on a candidate's local reputation. You've read it once and now you get to read it again: *An on-site inspection is essential!*[27]

Follow up on your recruiting efforts to ensure retention of those you have recruited. Maintain ongoing personal contact with the practices. Constantly endeavor to show you recognize the value of the practicing physician's time. And continue through newsletters, reports, and meetings to let the investigators know they are part of a team.

Get The Trials In Motion

On the one hand, you've been told repeatedly to get all your ducks in a row before you begin. On the other, you are most likely to lose physicians (and patients) who have signed up on paper but have not yet made an actual emotional commitment to the trials. Thus the majority of physician and patient recruitment should be performed only *after* the design process is completed and software development is well under way.

Recruitment of physicians and the initial recruitment of patients should be brief and intense, concentrated in a few short weeks. Ideally, training of the physician and his staff and appointment of a site coordinator should begin shortly thereafter. Physicians will begin to drop out or develop other interests if too much time elapses between recruitment and the start of the trials.

---

[27]Don't believe or don't want to believe that physicians can be corrupt? See Lock (1990) and Wells (1992).

PATIENT RECRUITMENT

Successful recruitment depends on developing a careful plan with multiple strategies, maintaining flexibility, establishing interim goals, and preparing to devote the necessary effort.[28]

Invariably, the number of patients actually recruited is many times less than the number predicted. Physicians tend to overestimate the amount of eligible patients they will treat during the course of the study, sometimes offering numbers 5–10 times in excess of what they might reasonably hope to achieve. Many investigators will recruit no patients at all, wasting the efforts you've put into training them and their staff and pocketing any setup monies you've provided. Worse, some investigators will recruit exactly one patient (or one less than the number of treatment arms), with the result that their efforts are (almost) unusable. ("Almost" because any adverse events at that site would still need to be reported.)

Rahman, Morita, Fukui, and Sakamoto (2004) find that the main reasons for physicians not entering patients are concern about the detrimental effects on the doctor-patient relationship, patients' refusal, complicated registration and follow-up procedures, and not feeling comfortable recruiting their own patients.

To obtain the number of subjects you want in the time period you've allotted you need to monitor the recruitment efforts of your investigators and engage in lengthy and costly recruiting efforts of your own.

Factors in Recruitment

Before going into the various methods for recruitment one might employ, let's first ask ourselves why a prospective subject might not enroll in our study. Four obvious reasons are that the subject

1. Doesn't know about the study
2. Doesn't want to be in the study
3. Doesn't satisfy the eligibility criteria
4. Is enrolled in a similar study

The first of these barriers can be addressed in three ways:

1. **Media campaigns**—radio and TV announcements, newspaper and magazine articles directed at the population of prospective patients
2. **Direct contact with all the physicians in a given area**
3. **Reinforcing the recruiting efforts of your study investigators**

---

[28]Friedman, Furberg, and DeMets (1996; p. 141).

All routes, not just the latter, should be utilized.

Understanding the factors underlying the decision to participate doesn't take a rocket scientist. Put yourself in the potential subject's place: Why might you be willing to give up part of your time and place yourself at risk to be part of a clinical study? Humanitarian concerns, perhaps? We all want to be part of something meaningful.

But we are most likely to participate when we perceive the possibility of a direct benefit to ourselves or to those we love. For example, in a study of pain-relieving agents, individuals who have suffered from headaches or whose close relatives have suffered are more likely to be volunteers.[29] In fact, today many individuals may deliberately seek out clinical trials in which they might participate (Metz et al., 2005). A resource for such individuals is provided by *http://www.veritasmedicine.com/*. See also the study of cancer patient recruitment by Sateren et al. (2002).

The ideal advertising campaign will let prospective patients know they can satisfy their own needs while helping others. Other factors that tend to attract volunteers are the promise of personal attention and care by specialists (Mattson, Curb and McArdle, 1985), money, and the lure of being part of something significant.

To increase participation in a study, you need to

- **Understand what the benefits are**
- **Increase the benefits**
- **Ensure that prospective study participants know about the benefits**

Importance of Planning

The importance of planning cannot be overestimated. You need to know whether other similar studies are in progress that might compete with yours for patients. A convenient registry of ongoing international (Australia, Britain, Canada, Hong Kong) clinical trials may be found at *http://www.controlled-trials.com/*. In the U.S. a similar registry may be found at *http://www.centerwatch.com/patient/trials.htm*.

I'd also recommend that you conduct trials of the various recruitment methods to see which is likely to be the most successful.

Tilley and Shorack (1990) found that typical problems that arise during recruitment include the following:

---

[29]But see Ellis et al. (1999).

- **Inadequate funding for screening**
- **Unwillingness of physicians to refer patients**
- **Overestimation of the prevalence of the condition**
- **Overly rigorous entry criteria**

All of these barriers to success can be addressed to a degree by careful planning and consistant monitoring of results. For example, to overcome the unwillingness of physicians to refer patients, consider holding an informative conference/cocktail party for local physicians in areas where recruitment is lagging. Computer-assisted data entry gives you the opportunity to continuously monitor recruitment and respond quickly.[30]

Ethical Considerations

Enrollment must be monitored on a continuous basis to forestall the tendency of the very few less than ethical physicians to enroll unsuitable subjects or to skip (or, more often, sidestep) informed consent. Ideally, eligibility forms should be reviewed on the day they are completed and before the start of the trial itself (the notable exception being when immediate intervention is dictated). Fortunately, computer-assisted data entry facilitates rapid review. But computerized analysis alone is not adequate. Frequent visits should be made routinely to each investigator's site.

A word of caution: Although investigators often rely successfully on referrals from potential subjects' personal physicians, Sugarman et al. (1999) warn that direct solicitation of subjects by their personal physician does not increase the recruitment rate and may be unethical.

Mass Recruiting

Mass recruiting efforts may be directed both toward the community at large and toward physician practice-based populations.

One way to reach the community at large is by providing free screening at health fairs, church groups and other organizations, and sports events. Other alternatives in common use include mass mailings with utility bills and newspaper and radio advertisements. No one best method exists. Given the innumerable specialized contacts required with any of these methods, I'd recommend employing a professional recruiting firm.

---

[30]You'll find a list of commercially available software for use in monitoring in the Appendix. Forecasting methods are described in Chapter 14.

Handberg-Thurmond et al. (1998) found that the highest yield was obtained by screening records of patients directly referred by a physician for possible study entry. Working through physicians, Margitic et al. (1999) found the self-administered office-based questionnaire to be the least costly strategy for one site ($14 per randomized participant), followed by patient mailing at another site ($58). The direct telephone contact method utilized at one site serving primarily a minority population yielded a cost per randomized participant of $80.

Mailings and media are effective when the target population is large and knowledgeable about the disease and treatment being investigated. The yield from mailings is greatest when individuals in the mailing list are familiar with both the research and the research center. An interpersonal approach is more effective than a media-based approach when the target population is small, unaware of their personal risk of the disease, or unfamiliar with research and research center (Resio, Baltch, and Smith, 2004).

Patient Retention

All your recruiting efforts will go for naught (and double your costs) if the patients you've recruited drop out of the study or do not comply with the protocol.

The three keys to patient retention are

- **Selecting the appropriate participants**
- **Optimizing the trial experience from the patient's point of view**
- **Monitoring compliance**

The more reasons a patient has for participating in a trial, the more likely he is to remain in compliance. Money alone won't cut it, at least not over an extended period. Although there has been extensive research in the area, no single set of demographic factors has proved to be consistent predictors of success. (See, for example, some of the articles in Haynes, Taylor, and Sackett, 1979, and in Shumaker, Schron, and Ockene, 1990.)

Keep the interval between screening and the actual onset of treatment to a minimum. Until the actual onset of treatment, prospective patients feel little or no loyalty to the study. Consciously or unconsciously they may have already forgotten (or may actually regret) their decision to enroll. When the delay is protracted, the prospective patient should be contacted and, if possible, rewarded during the interval to reinforce her commitment.

Ensure that the patient is fully informed (Sturdee, 2000) and that the directions he is provided with are unambiguous. Study physicians should be encouraged to spend ample time with each patient for this purpose. Your team should prepare and provide the physician with descriptive materials to be given the patient at the conclusion of an interview.

Physicians should be encouraged (and paid) to give all study patients VIP treatment: no long delays in crowded waiting rooms or being left for hours half-dressed in some isolated chamber. If a wait is necessary—surgeons do have emergencies—the site coordinator may have to spend time with the patient or make immediate alternate arrangements. In any event, the health provider, the site coordinator, and all members of the provider's staff who come in contact with the patient must be prepared to spend additional time to provide for the trial subject's need for assurance.

Not all of a patient's declared needs are genuine; some, from the health provider's point of view, are spurious. A major motivator for having a sponsor-paid coordinator at each site is to have someone to deal in a positive fashion with the overly garrulous, the overly demanding. We want not only the patient, but also the investigator and his staff, to remain committed throughout the study.

Ongoing Efforts

None of the preceding can be relied upon to ensure compliance unless you continuously monitor the investigators and prod them, if necessary, to submit scheduled follow-up reports. Again, computer-assisted data entry can only facilitate such monitoring.

Your staff can contribute to compliance in several additional ways:

- **Keep the protocol simple. One pill a day is preferable to three- or four-times-a-day regimens. Crossover designs, beloved by statisticians, will only confuse the participants if they entail changes in dosage schedules. Keep it simple.**
- **Provide special pill dispensers or automate injectibles so the patient has less to keep track of. Colorful reminder stickers, a watch that says "It's time to take your pill," and rewards for compliance are also of value.**
- **Consider preparing and distributing a newsletter to and for study subjects that will make them feel part of a team engaged in a worthwhile effort. The newsletter should be distributed on at least a quarterly basis (and more often if there is actual news). The contents of such a newsletter might include current statistics on the study's progress, profiles of study investigators, and reports gleaned from the media on the disease condition that is at the core of the study.**

Finally, you need to develop a method for monitoring patient compliance. Automated methods and pill counts are of dubious value. (See the texts cited earlier.) I recommend direct contact, via telephone, with each participant. Not that the information you gather will be any more reliable, but such calls serve the dual purpose of making the patient feel part of something important and thus more conscientious in compliance.

You may learn via telephone of adverse events: "I had to stop taking the pills because I was throwing up." Such responses should trigger calls from your staff to the subject's physician for further investigation. As the "blindness" of the treatment must be preserved, those making the calls on your behalf should not be aware of which treatment arm the patient was assigned to.

Run-In Period

Opinions differ on whether a run-in period should be used to identify and exclude patients who are unlikely to remain in compliance. During this period, best limited to three to six weeks before the start of the actual intervention, potential participants would be given either active medication or placebo and their compliance would be monitored. (See sidebar).

According to Friedman, Furburg, and DeMets (1996), the results have been almost uniformly positive—see, for example, Knipschild, Leffers, and Feinstein (1991) and Lang (1990). Although single-blind placebo run-ins are in common use today, Evans (2000) finds the practice ethically unjustified if they entail the withholding of medication. Milgrom et al. (1997) argue that run-ins have not yet been shown to be cost-effective and may endanger recruitment success.

Davis et al. (1995) put the hypothesis to the test by prescribing placebo for a three-week period before the start of their clinical trials but not using the results of this run-in period as an entry criterion. Of the 431 participants in their study, 66 (15%) who took less than 80% of the prescribed placebo or who failed to return their unused placebo pills were classified as poor run-in adherers. Poor run-in adherence was associated with lower educational attainment. At 3 and 6 months of follow-up, mean adherence was 89.3% and 83.4% among all participants. Exclusion of poor run-in adherers would have increased these means by one to two percent to 90.9% and 85.5%, respectively. Would a one to two percent gain in enrollment be worth the expense of those three extra weeks?

Run-in periods also can be used to exclude placebo responders and subjects who cannot tolerate or do not respond to active drug.

> **RUN-IN PERIOD**
>
> The following material is taken from the protocol for a study of colorectal adenoma chemoprevention using aspirin:
>
> "At 6 weeks, assess by telephone the patient's suitability for randomization based on compliance, motivation, and toxicity. If the patient appears suitable, telephone them again in 10 weeks. If the patient appears suitable at 10 weeks, proceed to randomization. If the patient is deemed not suitable at 6 or at 10 weeks, complete and submit the eligibility form stating the reason for withdrawal."

Pablos-Mendez, Barr, and Shea (1998) argue that the result of such use is to select a group of individuals who may differ markedly from patients undergoing active clinical management for this problem. However, after reviewing some 101 studies, Trivedi and Rush (1994) find that the use of a run-in period does not appear to enhance the drug/placebo differential.

Schechtman and Gordon (1993) find that run-in strategies are most likely to be cost-effective under the following conditions: 1) Per patient costs during the post-randomization as compared to the screening period are high; 2) poor compliance is associated with a substantial reduction in response to treatment; 3) the number of screened patients needed to identify a single eligible patient is small; 4) the run-in is inexpensive; 5) for most patients, the run-in compliance status is maintained after randomization; 6) many subjects excluded by the run-in are treatment intolerant or noncompliant to the extent that little or no treatment response is expected. Schechtman and Gordon find that run-ins are least cost-effective if their only purpose is to exclude ordinary partial compliers.

BUDGETS AND EXPENDITURES

Sweat the small stuff. Attorneys do it; so do CPAs. Don't just record major expenditures—air travel and outlays to advertising agencies—but track every phone call and the time your staff spends on it. Successful recruiting, and success is defined as retaining those you recruit, requires sustained effort. See Chapter 15.

FOR FURTHER INFORMATION

Agras WS; Bradford RH; Marshall GD, eds. (1992) Recruitment for clinical trials: the Lipid Research Clinics Coronary Primary Prevention Trial experience. Its implications for future trials. *Circulation* 66 (suppl IV): IV-1–IV-78.

Carey TS; Kinsinger L; Keyserling T; Harris R. (1996) Research in the community: recruiting and retaining practices. *J Community Health* 21:315–327.

Chadwick B; Treasure ET. (2005) Primary care research: difficulties recruiting preschool children to clinical trials. *Int J Paediatr Dent* 15(3):197–204.

Cramer JA. (1998) *Improving and Supporting Patient Recruitment In Clinical Trials Conducted by Academic Medical Centers.* Oak Brook IL: University HealthSystem Consortium.

Davis CE; Applegate WB; Gordon DJ; Curtis RC; McCormick M. (1995) An empirical evaluation of the placebo run-in. *Control Clin Trials* 16:41–50.

Donovan JL; Peters TJ; Noble S; Powell P; Gillatt D; Oliver SE; Lane JA; Neal DE; Hamdy FC; ProtecT Study Group. (2003) Who can best recruit to randomized trials? Randomized trial comparing surgeons and nurses recruiting patients to a trial of treatments for localized prostate cancer (the ProtecT study). *J Clin Epidemiol* 56:605–609.

Ellis PM; Dowsett SM; Butow PN; Tattersall MH. (1999) Attitudes to randomized clinical trials amongst out-patients attending a medical oncology clinic. *Health Expect* 2:33–43.

Evans M. (2000) Justified deception? The single blind placebo in drug research. *J Med Ethics* 26:188–193. (see also comment at 26:477)

Friedman LM; Furberg CD; DeMets DL. (1996) *Fundamentals of Clinical Trials*, 3rd Ed. St Louis, Mosby.

Gillum RF; Barsky AJ. (1974) Diagnosis and management of patient noncompliance. *JAMA* 228:1563–1567.

Gitanjali B; Raveendran R; Pandian DG; Sujindra S. (2003) Recruitment of subjects for clinical trials after informed consent: does gender and educational status make a difference? *J Postgrad Med* 49:109–113.

Haidich AB; Ioannidis JP. (2001) Determinants of patient recruitment in a multicenter clinical trials group: trends, seasonality and the effect of large studies. *BMC Med Res Methodol* 1:4.

Haidich AB; Ioannidis JP. (2003) Late-starter sites in randomized controlled trials. *J Clin Epidemiol* 56:408–415.

Handberg-Thurmond E; Baker A; Coglianese ME. et al. (1998) Identifying high yield sources of patients with coronary artery disease for clinical trials: lessons from the Asymptomatic Cardiac Ischemia Pilot (ACIP) experience. The ACIP Study Group. *Clin Cardiol* 21:176–182.

Haynes RB; Taylor DW; Sackett DL, eds. (1979). *Compliance in Health Care.* Baltimore: Johns Hopkins Press.

Hunninghake DB; Blaskowski TP, eds. (1987) Proceedings of the workshop on the recruitment experience in NHLBI-sponsored clinical trials. *Control Clin Trials* 8 (suppl).

Keith SJ. (2001) Evaluating characteristics of patient selection and dropout rates. *J Clin Psychiatry* 62 Suppl 9:11–14; discussion 15–16.

Knipschild P; Leffers P; Feinstein AR. (1991) The qualification period. *J Clin Epidemiol* 44:461–464.

Lang JM. (1990) The use of a run-in to enhance compliance. *Stat Med* 9:87–95.

Lock SP. (1990) Research fraud: discouraging the others. *BMJ* 301:1348.

Lung Health Study Research Group. (1993) The Lung Health Study: design of the trial and recruitment of participants. *Control Clin Trials* 14 (suppl).

Margitic S. et al. (1999) Challenges faced in recruiting patients from primary care practices into a physical activity intervention trial. *Prev Med* 29:277–286.

McBride PE; Massoth KM. et al. (1996) Recruitment of private practices for primary care research: experience in a preventive services clinical trial. *J Fam Pract* 43:389–395.

Metz JM; Coyle C; Hudson C; Hampshire M. (2005) An Internet-based cancer clinical trials matching resource. *J Med Internet Res* 7:e24.

Milgrom PM; Hujoel PP; Weinstein P; Holborow DW. (1997) Subject recruitment, retention, and compliance in clinical trials in periodontics. *Ann Periodontol* 2:64–74.

Pablos-Mendez A; Barr RG; Shea S. (1998) Run-in periods in randomized trials: implications for the application of results in clinical practice. *JAMA* 279:222–225. (See also comments in 279:1526–1527.)

Rahman M; Morita S; Fukui T; Sakamoto J. (2004) Physicians' reasons for not entering their patients in a randomized controlled trial in Japan. *Tohoku J Exp Med* 203:105–109.

Resio MA; Baltch AL; Smith RP. (2004) Mass mailing and telephone contact were effective in recruiting veterans into an antibiotic treatment randomized clinical trial. *J Clin Epidemiol* 57:1063–1070.

Ruffin MT 4th; Baron J. (2000) Recruiting subjects in cancer prevention and control studies. *J Cell Biochem Suppl* 34:80–83.

Sateren WB; Trimble EL; Abrams J; Brawley O; Breen N; Ford L; McCabe M; Kaplan R; Smith M; Ungerleider R; Christian MC. (2002) How sociodemographics, presence of oncology specialists, and hospital cancer programs affect accrual to cancer treatment trials. *J Clin Oncol* 20:2109–2117.

Schechtman KB; Gordon ME. (1993) A comprehensive algorithm for determining whether a run-in strategy will be a cost-effective design modification in a randomized clinical trial. *Stat Med* 12:111–128.

Schumaker SA; Schron EB; Ockene JK, eds. (1990) *Health Behavior Change.* New York: Springer.

Spilker B; Cramer JA. (1992) *Patient Recruitment in Clinical Trials.* New York: Raven.

Sturdee DW. (2000) The importance of patient education in improving compliance. *Climacteric* 3 Suppl 2:9–13.

Sugarman J; Regan K; Parker B; Bluman LG; Schildkraut J. (1999) Ethical ramifications of alternative means of recruiting research participants from cancer registries. *Cancer* 86:647–651.

Tilley BC; Shorack MA. (1990) Designing clinical trials of treatment for osteoporosis: recruitment and followup. *Calcif Tissue Int* 47:327–331.

Trivedi MH; Rush H. (1994) Does a placebo run-in or a placebo treatment cell affect the efficacy of antidepressant medications? *Neuropsychopharmacology* 11:33–43 (with comments in 15:105, 107).

Weiner DL; Butte AJ; Hibberd PL; Fleisher GR. (2003) Computerized recruiting for clinical trials in real time. *Ann Emerg Med* 41:242–246.

Wells F. (1992) Fraud and misconduct in clinical research: is it prejudicial to patient safety? *Adverse Drug React Toxicol Rev* 11:241–255.

Chapter 10
Computer-Assisted Data Entry

Electronic Case Report Form (e-CRF) means an auditable electronic record designed to record information required by the clinical trial protocol to be reported to the sponsor on each trial subject.
Guidance For Industry, Computerized Systems Used In Clinical Trials[31]

Computer-assisted data entry offers at least six advantages over paper case report forms:

- **Immediate detection and correction of errors.** Mistakes such as typographical errors and misplaced decimal points are detected and corrected at the time of entry. No data are lost as a result of lapses in memory.
- **Reduced sources of error.** Eliminating the need to recode and reenter case report forms eliminates two potential sources of error. There is a corresponding reduction in costs.
- **Open ended.** If inspection of the "other" category reveals that "protein imbalance" is being written in with a relatively high frequency, then "protein imbalance" can be added to the options on the pull-down menu. Printed case report forms are fixed, lifeless.
- **Quality control.** Even the best-designed forms can contain ambiguities just as even the best-designed trials can have unexpected consequences. Measuring devices can go out of tolerance. By tabulating and monitoring the information as it is collected, problems at some or all of the sites can be detected and corrected early on.
- **Improved investigator relations.** If a trend is detected, particularly if it only involves one or two sites, it can be difficult to communi-

---

[31] http://www.fda.gov/ora/compliance_ref/bimo/ffinalcct.pdf.

A Manager's Guide to the Design and Conduct of Clinical Trials, by Phillip I. Good
Copyright ©2006 John Wiley & Sons, Inc.

cate the need for modification of procedures without offending some investigators. Let the clinical research monitor (CRM) and the investigator jointly blame the software.

- Ease of access. Generally, the same software that simplifies data entry makes it easy for the non-computer professional to access and display the result. (We expand on this point in Chapter 11) Both your staff and the regulatory agency will have earlier access to trial data compared with paper CRFs.
- Many regulatory agencies such as the FDA now accept and even prefer electronic submissions (also known as e-subs or CANDAs), thus doing away with the need to manage or store paper case report forms. If paper forms are required, they are readily produced. And if a paper form turns up missing, it is easily regenerated from the electronic record and submitted to the investigator for signature. (Security procedures for electronic records are discussed in Chapter 11, also.)

Implementation of computer-assisted entry involves three steps:

1. Developing and testing the data entry software
2. Training medical and paramedical personnel in the software's use
3. Monitoring the quality of the data.

We discuss the first two of these steps in the following sections, and the last step in Chapters 13 and 14.

PRE-DATA SCREEN DEVELOPMENT CHECKLIST

All required data have been grouped by the individual who will collect the data (patient, front-office person, nurse, physician) and the time at which it will be collected (initial screen, baseline, 1-week follow-up).

For each data item, the units and acceptable range have been specified. See Table 10.1.

DEVELOP THE DATA ENTRY SOFTWARE

The first steps in software development are to

- Decide which software product to use to develop the data-entry screens (A list of commercially available software is provided in the Appendix.)

TABLE 10.1 Data Specifications Table

Item	Group	Units	Question if	Reject unless
Year of birth	Bp	Year		17 < (Current year − Birth year) < 81
Diastolic pressure	B,Fn	mmHg	DP < 50 or DP > 110	30 < DP < systolic pressure

- Organize the required information into functional groups using the CDISC guidelines
- Prepare a flow or Gant chart for the development process

The responsibility for choosing the development languages for data entry, data management, and data analysis is normally divided among the lead developer, the data manager, and the statistician. The project manager may be called upon to resolve conflicts not only among the members of this committee but with other units of the corporation.

The lists of required information and the associated questions prepared by the design committee should be divided into functional groups. Each group consists of a set of questions that will be answered at the same time by the same individual.

These groupings should parallel the time line you developed during the design phase.

- **Eligibility**
    - **Questions to determine eligibility for inclusion in the study**
    - **Patient demographics including risk factors**
- **Baseline**
    - **Evaluation of condition**
    - **Laboratory values**
    - **Special studies (e.g., angiogram)**
    - **Concurrent medications**
- **Intervention data**
- **Hospital summary (if applicable)**
- **Follow-up**
    - **Evaluation of condition (subjective, objective)**
    - **Events during interval**
    - **Laboratory values**
    - **Special studies (e.g., angiogram)**
    - **Concurrent medications**
- **Adverse event reports**
    - **Nature of event**
    - **Hospital summary, special studies, autopsy (when applicable)**
- **Protocol deviation**

Each type of special study will require its own set of data entry screens. Normally, one of the CRMs will oversee preparation of these groupings.

The lead developer is responsible for preparing a flow or Gant chart for the development process. This chart will include the work assignments for each individual assigned to the project. I recommend that each functional group be the responsibility of a single developer working in tandem with a single CRM. Between them they will work out the context and sequencing of the screens needed to record their portion of the data.

One natural ordering of tasks follows the sequence in which the screens will be completed at the study centers. Those screens devoted to eligibility determination that contain the inclusion and exclusion criteria should be developed first, followed by the screens that will contain the baseline clinical information, risk factors, medical history, physical assessment, current medications, and baseline laboratory values. For the reasons outlined in Chapter 7, these screens should already be tested and in the hands of the investigators while the last of the follow-up, adverse event, and patient contact forms are still undergoing development.

Avoid Predefined Groupings in Responses

Avoid the use of predefined groups in forms.

For example, rather than asking the patients to classify their smoking habit as in Smoker (never, quit over 1 month, $<\frac{1}{2}$ pk/day, $\frac{1}{2}$ to 1 pk/day, >1 pk/day), have them enter the number of years they've smoked, their average pack per day consumption, and whether they are current smokers.

Rather than classifying cholesterol levels as in Hypercholesterolemia (<200 mg/dl, 200 to 235 mg/dl, requires medication), enter the exact measurement of cholesterol level obtained in baseline screening.

Avoiding predefined groupings gives us much greater flexibility and allows us to use metric variables rather than categorical ones, paving the way for the use of more sensitive statistics. We can measure exposure to cigarette smoke in pack years or we can classify and group smokers in various different ways for different report purposes after the data have been collected., for example, never, quit over 2 months, $<\frac{3}{4}$ pk/day, $\frac{3}{4}$ to 2 pk/day, >2 pk/day.

SCREEN DEVELOPMENT

In computer-aided data entry, the computer's screen, approximately 80 characters wide by 24 lines, plays the role that printed case report forms once did. There is no need to copy or ape the printed form. The focus should be on making effective use of the screen. For example, rather than trying to cram a single form onto a single

> **SAMPLE FORM SPECIFICATIONS**
>
> Form: Risk Factors 1
> To be completed at: Baseline patient interview
> To be completed by: Examining nurse
>
> FIELDS
> Patient Name (last, first, MI)
> Patient ID (display only)
> Patient address and telephone number (display/update)
>
> Does patient have significant GI bleeding (yes/no)?
> Does patient have peripheral vascular disease (yes/no)?
>
> Diabetes mellitus (none, treated with exercise diet alone, oral hypoglycemics, insulin)
> Current smoker (yes/no)
> Smoker (current or past)   _____number of years; _____number packs per day
>
> Hypertension (<90 mmHg, 90–100 mmHg, requires medication)
> Has patient had a previous myocardial infarction? (yes/no)
> (skip next fields if no)   date of most recent MI
>   Q-wave (yes/no/unknown)
>
> Weight (specify kg or lb) (question if not 100 to 280) (refuse if not 80 to 325)
>
> Specifications prepared by: L Moore 19 Nov 2002
> Specifications approved by: JR Moon 8 Dec 2002

screen, the layout should be dictated by the comfort and convenience of the potential user. Small type and crowded screens should be avoided.

Although the developer is responsible for the layout, the CRM should dictate the sequencing of questions and screens based on his or her knowledge of how the potential user (nurse, technician, specialist) is likely to acquire the information. The CRM is also responsible for filling in any gaps left by the design committee when they specified the range of permissible answers for each question.

An example would be a question on smoking habits. To the selection, "a pack a day," "two packs per day," "more than two packs," the CRM might need to add, "less than a pack per day." (Though, as

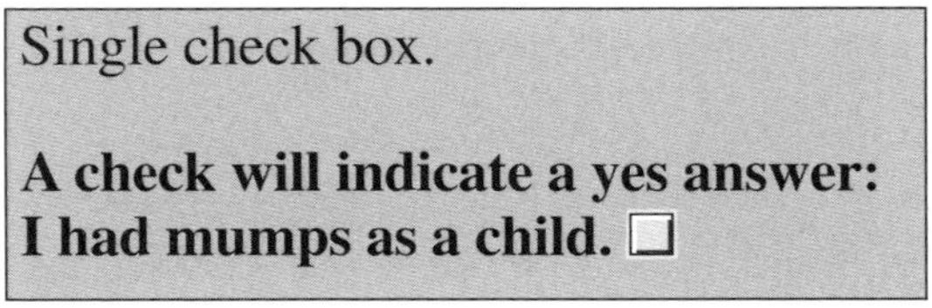

> Single check box.
>
> **A check will indicate a yes answer:
> I had mumps as a child.** ☐

FIGURE 10.1a

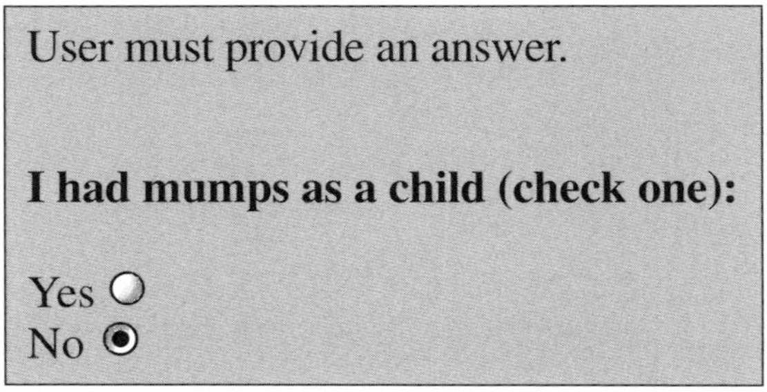

> User must provide an answer.
>
> **I had mumps as a child (check one):**
>
> Yes ○
> No ⦿

FIGURE 10.1b

already noted, this question would be better phrased as How many packs a week do you smoke?")

Each question is represented on the screen by one of three formats, the radio button and pull-down menu for multiple-choice questions and the type-and-verify field for numeric responses.

Radio Button

The radio button depicted in Figure 10.1a is recommended when there are only a few options and only one option may be selected. All alternatives should be displayed. A single check "yes" button as in Figure 10.1a is not acceptable. Figure 10.1b shows the correct approach. If neither a "yes" nor a "no" is checked, the cursor will not advance to the next question.

What if the respondent doesn't know or doesn't remember the answer? Then a third option should be incorporated as in Figure 10.1c. Skipping the question cannot be permitted, for a major objective of computer-assisted data entry is the elimination of missing data and the need for extensive time-consuming follow-up.

Figure 10.1d illustrates the use of graphics and layout options to create a user-friendly design for the data entry screen.

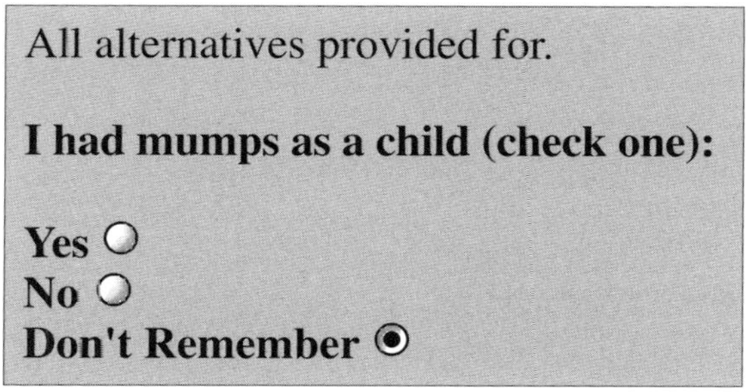

> All alternatives provided for.
>
> **I had mumps as a child (check one):**
>
> Yes ○
> No ○
> **Don't Remember** ●

FIGURE 10.1c

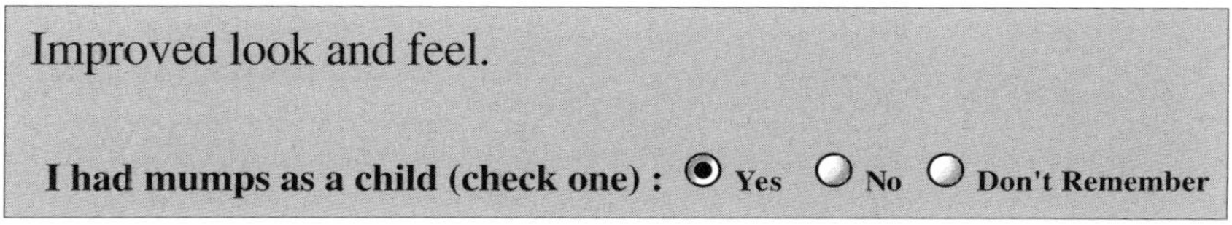

> Improved look and feel.
>
> **I had mumps as a child (check one) :** ● Yes   ○ No   ○ Don't Remember

FIGURE 10.1d

Pull-Down Menus

Pull-down or pop-up menus are of two types, those that permit only a single selection from a menu of choices and those that permit multiple selections. The type of permission needs to be specified in advance by the forms design committee.

Note in Figure 10.2 that not all the choices are displayed but can be accessed by scrolling through the pull-down menu using the side arrows. Hopefully, a field labeled "other" is in the part of the menu we can't see.

Type and Verify

The type and verify field (Fig. 10.3) is used for two types of data: measurements and comments such as "Other risk factors include. . . ." A set of bounds needs to be specified for each measurement that will be entered in a type-and-verify field. Actually, two sets of bounds need to be specified: The first set rules out the impossible, a negative value of cholesterol, for example. If an impossible value is displayed, the following message would appear on the screen: "A negative value is not possible, please reenter the value. Press enter to continue." When the user presses the enter key, the cursor returns to the field where the erroneous entry was made so that data can be reentered.

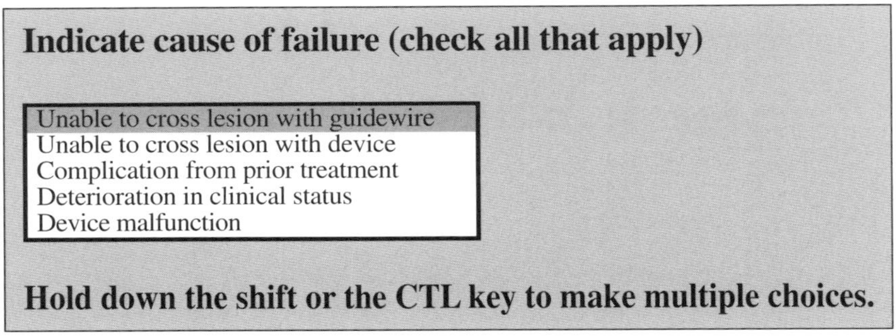

Indicate cause of failure (check all that apply)

Unable to cross lesion with guidewire
Unable to cross lesion with device
Complication from prior treatment
Deterioration in clinical status
Device malfunction

Hold down the shift or the CTL key to make multiple choices.

FIGURE 10.2

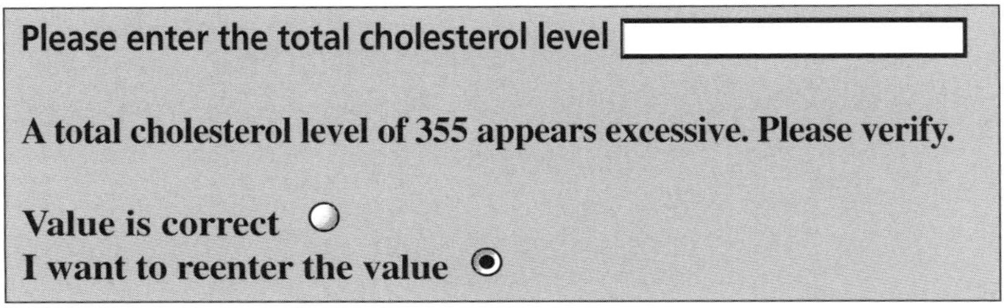

Please enter the total cholesterol level [   ]

A total cholesterol level of 355 appears excessive. Please verify.

Value is correct ○
I want to reenter the value ●

FIGURE 10.3

The second set of bounds delineates so-called "normal" values, a total cholesterol level of more than 100 or less than 250, for example. Checking a "yes" would confirm the entry; checking a "no" would return the cursor to the field where the erroneous entry was made.

When the Entries Are Completed

After each screen is processed, a summary of the entries is displayed as in Figure 10.4 along with the message "Are these entries correct, "Yes or No?" A "yes" answer results in storing the entries in a file on disk and advancing the display to the next screen. A "no" answer returns the display to the just-completed screen so that corrections can be made.

Completing and accepting the last screen in a functional group triggers a printout of the completed case report form.

> **GUARANTEEING FAILURE**
>
> A sure way to guarantee failure is with bizarre keypunch instructions. Bumbling's printed case report form listed 9 possible adverse events (including an "other" category). Thus question 17.4 was Myocardial infarction, yes or no, question 17.5 was Stroke, yes or no, and so forth. The secret to analyzing the data was to realize that all 9 questions had been encoded to a single field using a total of 12 codes, listed—by the time I caught up with the ill-fated project—only on a faded handwritten piece of paper.
>
> To discourage casual users from attempting to scan the database by eye, Bumbling made sure a different set of codes would be used on each new form. While an atherectomy might be coded as a 420 on the adverse event form under the heading "action taken," when the atherectomy was actually performed it would be coded on the repeat revascularization form as a 511.
>
> Confused? So was everyone connected with the project.

Patient Risk Factors

Rhoda N. Morganstern
Born 26 Dec 1948
5'6" 155lbs Mdm Frame
Female multipara postmenopausal
No significant GI Bleeding
No peripheral vascular disease
Former smoker, quit over one year
No hypercholesterolemia
Hypertension, medication not required

Is this information correct?

Yes ○
No ◉

FIGURE 10.4

> **CODING FOR CHAOS**
>
> Bumbling Pharmaceutical's Information Services Director had joined the company in an era when expanding memory was done in chunks of kilobytes rather than megabytes and a large hard disk was one that held 10 megabytes instead of 5. Determined to save computer memory, he ruled that information should be coded whenever possible.
>
> The original printed case report form had provided for separate entries of each of half a dozen risk factors, with each factor further broken down into subcategories. Smoking history, for example, was broken down into "never smoked," "former smoker," and "current smoker." In the course of recoding the data, each category was assigned a separate numeric value so that "never smoked" was coded as 000 and "former smoker" as 021. All the "no's" on the form were assigned the same value of 000. The results were disastrous.
>
> The designers of the form had assumed that a 000 would appear on the completed form only if the patient answered "no" to all questions. But they had neglected the possibility of missing data. If the examining physician omitted to record whether or not the patient had diabetes, and checked "no" to all the other questions, a 000 appeared in the database, implying that the patient did not have diabetes even though quite the opposite might be true.

Audit Trail

One ought to have as much or more confidence in the data derived from computerized systems as in data originally in paper form. Some guiding principles for maintaining data integrity and a clear audit trail where computerized systems are being used to create, modify, maintain, archive, retrieve, or transmit clinical data may be downloaded from *http://www.fda.gov/ora/compliance_ref/bimo/ffinalcct.htm*.

ELECTRONIC DATA CAPTURE

Electronic Case Report Forms (e-CRF) are just one facet of electronic data capture (EDC). The others include

- **Direct data acquisition from laboratory instruments**
- **Handheld devices that allow patients and their caretakers to enter symptom/treatment data electronically accompanied by an automatic time-date stamp**

The only essential information that continues to elude EDC is *interpretation*, for example, "Tissue is malignant," "EKG reveals a myocardial infarction," "Spot on the mammogram is a cyst," "Adverse event is treatment related." Interpretations must be separately entered into a clinical database.

DATA STORAGE: CDISC GUIDELINES

In naming variables and formatting them for storage, we strongly recommend that you adhere to CDISC guidelines. The Clinical Data Interchange Standards

- **Speed up form preparation**
- **Help ensure completeness**
- **ODM facilitates data storage and retrieval**
- **Facilitate combination of data from diverse corporate entities**
- **Speed up the regulatory process**

The CDISC Submission Metadata Model was created to help ensure that the supporting metadata for submission datasets should meet the following objectives:

- **Provide regulatory agency reviewers with clear descriptions of the usage, structure, contents and attributes of all data sets and variables**
- **Allow reviewers to replicate most analyses, tables, graphs, and listings with minimal or no transformations, joins, or merges**
- **Enable reviewers to easily view and subset the data used to generate any analysis, table, graph, or listing without complex programming.**

The Model does not address specific content issues such as how to populate individual data sets for a particular study. The Model will guide you toward certain common conventions that, hopefully, should provide greater consistency and uniformity among all future submissions. The Model helps ensure that those data domains, elements, and attributes that are common to all submissions will be represented in the same manner in every case.

CDISC is a work in progress. For example, partial dates (August 2003 rather than 11 August 2003) are not provided for in the current version.

Descriptions of data fields and acceptable ranges are available in spreadsheet format at *http://www.cdisc.org/pdf/ SubmissionMetadataModelV2.pdf*. For example:

FIELD NAME	REQD	SAS VARIABLE NAME	DEFAULT REPRE- SENTATION	MAX LEN	DATA TYPE	EXPLANATION
Site Level						
Site ID or Number	Yes	SITEID	(none)	20	Text	The ID of the site.
Investigator Level						
Investigator ID or Number	No	INVID	(none)	20	Text	The ID of the investigator.
Investigator Name	No	INVNAM	(none)	80	Text	The name of the investigator.
Subject Level						
Screen ID or Number	Cond.	SCRNNUM	(none)	20	Text	The ID of the subject *before* randomization.
Subject Date Of Birth	No	BRTHDTM	YYYY-MM-DD	10	Text	The date of birth of the subject.

FIELD NAME	REQD FIELD?	SAS VARIABLE NAME	DEFAULT	MAX LEN	DATA TYPE	CODELIST
Subject Sex	No	SEX	(none)	1	Text	HL7 Gender Vocabulary Domain
Subject Sex Code List ID	No	SEXCD	(none)	40	Text	
Subject Race	No	RACE	(none)	20	Text	HL7 Race Vocabulary Domain
Subject Race Code List ID	No	RACECD	(none)	40	Text	
Subject Age Lower Limit	Yes	AGELO	(none)	3	Numeric	(none)
Subject Age Upper Limit	Yes	AGEHI	(none)	3	Numeric	(none)
Subject Age Units	Yes	AGEU	(none)	1	Text	(none)
Medical Condition	No	MEDCND	(none)	80	Text	(none)

As the following example illustrates, sample data are provided for test purposes. In short, with so much of the work done for you, adherence to CDISC standards will prove both timesaving and effective for data storage and transmission for review.

```
<?xml version="1.0" encoding="ISO-8859-1" ?>
- <!—
  CDISC Lab Model: Sample Output File
  —>
```

```xml
- <!--
  Not for Production Use
  -->
- <GTP ModelVersion="01-0-01" CreationDateTime=
  "2003-08-07T14:09:44-05:00">
    <TransmissionSource ID="A1234" Name="Central
      Lab ABC" />
  - <Study ID="CDISC Test 1" Name="CDISC Test 1"
    TransmissionType="C">
    - <Site ID="11">
      - <Investigator ID="11" Name="John Smith,
        M.D.">
        - <Subject>
          <ScreenID>8222</ScreenID>
          <Sex Value="M" CodeListID="HL7 V2.5
            Gender Vocabulary Domain" />
          <Confidential Initials="ABC"
            Birthdate="1968-08-12" />
        - <Visit ID="01" Name="Screen" Type="S">
          - <Accession ID="C434382"
            LastActiveDateTime="2001-05-
            10T11:34:50-05:00">
            <CentralLab ID="C1234" Name="Central
              Lab ABC" />
            - <BaseSpecimen ID="2">
              <SpecimenCollection
                ActualCollectionDateTime="2001-05-
                09T10:55:00-05:00" />
              <SpecimenTransport
                ReceivedDateTime="2001-05-
                10T06:25:00-05:00" />
              <SpecimenMaterial ID="SER"
                Name="Serum" CodeListID="HL7 V2.5
                0070 Specimen Source Table" />
              <SubjectAtCollection
                AgeAtCollection="32" AgeUnits="Y" />
              - <BaseBattery ID="RC3266"
                Name="CHEMISTRY">
                - <BaseTest Status="D" TestType="S">
                  <PerformingLab ID="L1234"
                    Name="Central Lab ABC - Chicago
                    NA" />
```

```
            <LabTest ID="RCT1" Name="Total
              Bilirubin" />
            <LOINCTestCode Value="14631-6"
              CodeListID="LOINC V3.7" />
        ‒  <BaseResult
              ReportedResultStatus="F"
              ReportedDateTime="2001-05-
              10T04:58:10-05:00">
            ‒  <SingleResult ResultClass="R"
                  ResultType="N">
                <TextResult Value="9" />
                <NumericResult Value="9"
                  Precision="" />
                <ResultReferenceRange
                  ReferenceRangeLow="3"
                  ReferenceRangeHigh="21" />
                <ResultUnits Value="umol/L"
                  CodeListID="ISO 1000" />
            </SingleResult>
```

TESTING

Testing is the responsibility of every team member and not just the testing department. Quality should be built in from the start. If multiple developers are employed, frequent meetings are necessary to ensure the developers use common naming and programming conventions. Each screen should be tested separately by its developer, then tested again by the developer as part of the larger integrated package before the program is turned over to the testing group to repeat the entire process.

The purpose of testing is twofold. The first purpose is to ensure the program does what it is supposed to do: If an 11.6 is entered from the keyboard, 11.6 should be recorded in the file and not 11.8 or 116. A cholesterol level of 250 should trigger a warning message as shown in Figure 10.3. A user should not be able to advance to the next screen of a series without filling in answers to all the questions on the screen she is currently viewing.

The second purpose of testing is to ensure that the program does *not* do what it is *not* supposed to do. If a cholesterol level of 2500 or 2.5 is typed in, it should not be entered into the file. And, most important, a doctor or nurse should never find herself staring at a screen that displays the following:

```
DataEntry32 caused an invalid page fault in
module MFC42.DLL at 015f:5f4040fd.
Registers:
EAX = 00000000 CS = 015f EIP = 5f4040fd EFLGS = 00010246
EBX = 00000000 SS = 0167 ESP = 007cf880 EBP = 008f2870
ECX = 5f4d1b4c DS = 0167 ESI = 007cf8a0 FS = 1147
EDX = 00000006 ES = 0167 EDI = 008f2504 GS = 0000
Bytes at CS:EIP:
83 78 f4 00 0f 8c 7c 7b 05 00 8b ce e8 6b f8 ff
Stack dump:
00000000 008f33a8 0045f8ca 008f2504 007cfb40
007ec8dc 008f3130 008f3130
5f4d1b58 008f2870 00000005 008f3130 008f3130
007cf8a8 007cf944 007cf944
```

No, I don't know what these numbers mean—does anyone?—but I know that once I see a display like this, I can wave goodbye to all the work I've done on the computer for the past hour or so. All the bugs should—no, must—be removed from your data entry programs before they reach your investigators.

Formal Testing

Formal testing generally falls into two phases: fully automated and hands-on. The primary automated testing tool is a screen-capture utility such as AQTest, SQA Test, Silktest, and WinRunner. These utilities emulate the process a human user goes through in entering data from the keyboard, doing so at ten times the speed and with no lapse in attention when the same test must be repeated over and over again with minor modifications. Testing tools work in three stages:

First, they make a record of the objects—radio buttons and pop-up menus that appear on the computer screen.

Second, they record the keystrokes their users make. If the user goes to the first question and checks a "no," they record that. If he types in 11.6 in answer to the next question, they record that. When this record is played back, each and every keystroke and mouse movement of the user is repeated.

The resulting recording can be displayed by the test program developer as a series of readily modified instructions to the computer. A standard modification consists of embedding the instructions in a loop so that the first time thorough the loop, the number 11.6 is entered, on the next occasion, 0.116, and on the next, 1160.

The reasoning behind this type of loop is that a well-designed testing program will use not only the type of data that is desired, but also the type that is unwanted, such as entries that exceed the pre-programmed bounds, leave some fields incomplete, and so forth.

Once such a test is developed, performing the automated test—the third stage—is as easy as pressing a button and requires an equal level of skill. A log of the test results is produced automatically and provides a permanent record of success or failure.

A further advantage of using a screen-capture utility comes when it is necessary to modify a screen by adding, deleting, or modifying any of the questions that appear on it. Once similar modifications to the testing program are completed, it is ready to loop through the test again and again, a thousand times or more if necessary.

Stress Testing

Automated testing suffers from the same weakness as the original programming process: the inability to foresee all that a naive computer user is liable to do in practice.

You may recall the climatic scene in the film "Good Will Hunting" in which Robin Williams playing the part of a psychiatrist tries to persuade an anxious Matt Damon that he is not really responsible for the abuse he suffered as a child. Matt keeps saying over and over that he knows he is not responsible, but it is obvious that on a deeper level he believes quite the opposite. Most of us are the same way about computers. If we see a message that says there is a program failure, we blame it on ourselves and try to avoid all contact with that program in the future. The result of such reactions in the case of a clinical trial will be to interfere with, interrupt, and, in some cases, sabotage data collection.

The purpose of stress testing a program before releasing it for use is to detect all problems in a setting where there is little or no risk of turning off potential users. Stress testing may follow a script or may be a totally ad hoc process. A non-computer professional should perform the test, ideally someone with a background similar to that of those who will be doing the data entry at the investigators' sites.

As the CRMs will be responsible for training in data entry, and must master use of the data entry screens, I recommend that the CRMs be used for the final stages of testing so they can combine the latter task with the former.

Warning: The project leader may need to get involved if a CRM reports that testing is uncovering an unusually large number of errors. A meeting of the development and testing teams should be called to ensure the project is brought back on course.

The effort preceding computer-assisted data entry is time consuming, but it is still only a fraction of the time that will be wasted if an inferior data entry process is allowed to slip by.

TRAINING

The CRM is responsible for training all the individuals—physicians, nurses, secretaries, and technicians—who will be entering the data. Thus she needs to be thoroughly familiar with the data entry process before training begins.

The training can be accomplished either in individual or in group training sessions. The normal sequence is to conduct training on a trial basis at one or two sites, then to give one or two group training sessions, and then to follow up with individual sessions for those sites who missed the group sessions along with those sites that request additional attention.

A similar strategy may need to be followed at each site, with training being given initially to one or two key individuals, followed by training for all those who might have access to the computer during the trials.

I recommend that the CRM pay an initial visit to each site accompanied by the person or persons responsible for installing the computer and the data entry software. The computer and software should be brought with them rather than sent on ahead. The idea being to avoid improper or incomplete installations and to ensure that the computer is placed where it can be used conveniently during the course of a patient examination or reading.[32]

The training phase is never really over, as testing site personnel will continue to come and go throughout the course of a lengthy trial. Part of the monitoring process discussed in Chapter 13 consists of a review of the data entry procedures at each site.

Reminder

Training for data entry is just part of an overall training program that

---

[32] Yes, sites have been known to rebel at such instrusions; it is far better to weed out and replace such sites at this stage rather than after the trials have started.

also encompasses patient recruitment and retention. The CRM needs to sit down with the principal investigator and coordinator at each site to ensure a mutual understanding of recruitment guidelines and patient handling. After such discussions, each site coordinator should be asked to submit a locally developed protocol for all phases of patient treatment with particular emphasis on contact and follow-up. As we discussed in Chapter 9, the objective of greater patient retention is best achieved by providing the patient with a positive reinforcing experience during each patient visit. Prolonged stays in waiting rooms or half-undressed in some isolated inside chamber do not qualify as "positive." (I hope my own physician is paying some attention to this.) Nor should the actual physician-patient contact appear rushed or hurried. VIP treatment is required for optimal patient retention. Study physicians and staff need to understand that such treatment is part of the commitment they've made.

SUPPORT

They've plopped a new computer on your desk along with software you've never seen before. You had a two-day training session (from which you had to miss 4 hours to take care of an emergency), and now you're on your own. Wouldn't you like to have a phone number to call just in case? A phone number where people will be on hand to answer when you need them regardless of differences in time zones?

SUPPORT IS ESSENTIAL

"Electronic clinical trials put very few technology demands on a user, and sites are usually unaware of the complexity of the underlying technology. Sites rightly expect that the technology will work when they need it and that it will not interfere with the core site functions of patient care and data collection and cleaning. While many sites have no problems running an EDC study, if technical issues develop, the sites have little or no access to the type of support they require to resolve these difficulties. Consequently, it is frequently the research staff that must take time away from their clinical tasks to work with the EDC vendor to resolve problems. The lack of local technology support and the ensuing technical demands placed on the site users are potentially serious obstacles to the acceptance of electronic clinical trials. In the long term, this problem will be alleviated as the proportion of electronic trials run at sites increases and the sites develop or outsource a local support infrastructure. EDC vendors and sponsors must carefully survey the technical support abilities of sites and, if they are insufficient, then make arrangements to either directly or indirectly provide onsite technical support."—J. Larus, PharmaLinkFHI

Now you've seen things from the investigator's point of view, you know that a hotline needs to be part of the data entry process. Ever have the experience of being told to call back the next day because the person on the other end of the line could only answer simple questions? When you set up your hotline, staff it with knowledgeable personnel.

BUDGETS AND EXPENDITURES

The budget for off-the-shelf hardware and software is firmed up during this phase.

I recommend the use of separate time codes to distinguish productive from nonproductive time. Delays in the arrival of hardware and software often leave programmers sitting on their hands. Similar delays arise when CRMs aren't available to answer questions. Information concerning the impact of delays is essential during posttrial review. See Chapter 15.

FOR FURTHER INFORMATION

Read articles and sign up for free newsletter on issues in electronic data capture at *http://www.phaseforward.com/*

A guide to *eClinical Trials: Planning and Implementation* may be ordered from *http://Centerwatch.com*.

Bassion S. (2002) Toward a laboratory data interchange standard for clinical trials. *Clin Chem* 48:2290–2292

Marquez LO; Stewart H. (2005) Improving medical imaging report turn-around times: the role of technology. *Radiol Manage* 27:26–31.

Verweij J; Nielsen OS; Therasse P; van Oosterom AT. (1997) The use of a systemic therapy checklist improves the quality of data acquisition and recording in multicentre trials. A study of the EORTC Soft Tissue and Bone Sarcoma Group. *Eur J Cancer* 33:1045–1049.

Chapter 11
Data Management

THIS CHAPTER IS DEVOTED TO DATA MANAGEMENT, not so that you can become an expert in the area, but so that you will understand the range of choices and be able to hold your own in discussions with "experts" from accounting and information systems (to say nothing of other executives who may have fallen under the spell of a salesperson). Three issues are discussed:

1. Choice of data management software and the options available to you
2. Transfer of data from data entry to data storage and from data storage to your report generating and statistical analysis software
3. Maintaining the security and integrity of your data

OPTIONS

Flat Files

Many managers would feel more comfortable if clinical data could be stored and viewed in a format with which they are already familiar, an Excel spreadsheet, for example (see Fig. 11.1). At first glance, the spreadsheet format seems ideal: each row constitutes a different patient record, and each column a different field or variable. But as we start to fill in a mockup of our spreadsheet, two difficulties arise: First, as the number of columns exceeds the width of the screen, we may easily forget just where a particular data item is located; second, as the trial continues, we begin to accumulate multiple records for each patient—pretreatment or baseline, one-week

---

A Manager's Guide to the Design and Conduct of Clinical Trials, by Phillip I. Good
Copyright ©2006 John Wiley & Sons, Inc.

	A	B	C	D	E	F
1						Recurrent Ischemia
2	PATID	EVENT	PAGE	Date	Adverse Event	R2/R3
3	002-1121	1MON		8/15/98	FATIGUE	
4	002-1121	6MON		8/15/98	FATIGUE	
5	002-1122	6MON	117_HOSP	1/31/99	EPIGASTRIC PAIN	
6	002-1122	YEAR		8/26/99	UTI, HEMATURIA	
7	002-1124	2WEK		9/30/98	Allergic Reaction	

FIGURE 11.1 Spreadsheet as an Example of a Flat File.

follow-up, one-month follow-up, and, so forth. Will we run out of space?

The first of these difficulties is correctable, not by Excel, but by a more advanced flat file manager that would allow us to search for columns by name.

The second difficulty presents more of a challenge, particularly when the different follow-ups involve different examinations and thus different sets of variables. Although each patient's baseline record contains a host of information including demographic variables, baseline data, and laboratory values, the various follow-ups may contain only a few data items. On the other hand, the adverse event record contains many items that are not in the baseline record. When we create a column for each variable that "might" occur, the result is a worksheet made up primarily of space-consuming blank entries.

Obviously, we will need several spreadsheets to store our data, perhaps one for each record type or each set of screens. But then how are we to link them in such a way that we can search and retrieve information from several worksheets at a time? Moreover, as the number and size of our worksheets grows, access times increase and corrections become more difficult.

Suppose a follow-up exam file includes fields for the date, patient name, patient ID, patient address, plus the observations on that patient on that date. Each record must repeat the name, ID, and address of the patient, increasing the amount of storage required and perhaps doubling or even tripling the time required for data retrieval.

A ten-column spreadsheet with 2000 entries requires about 200 Kbytes of storage and takes only a few seconds to sort. But a typical clinical database requires 200,000 Kbytes of storage and 1000 to 10,000 seconds to sort if the sorting methods used by Excel (one of the fastest spreadsheets) were employed.

If the patient's address changes, it will have to be changed in multiple locations or risk irresolvable inconsistencies. If the patient's name is spelled differently in different places (e.g., Phil Good, Phillip Good) then we may fail to retrieve all the necessary records.

In summary, a flat file database like a spreadsheet contains only one record structure, many of whose fields will be empty. Access to data is done in a sequential manner; access times are slow because the entire file must be scanned to locate the desired data. Complex queries—"How many patients who were heavy smokers suffered non-Q-wave MIs during the first three months after the stent was implanted?"—are virtually impossible as there are no links between separate records.

Other problems with a flat file database include data redundancy, the difficulty of locating and updating records as the file size increases, and the near impossibility of maintaining data integrity.[33] When the regulatory agency makes unexpected requests, will we be able to respond quickly?

Hierarchical Databases

The traditional answer to some of these issues was the hierarchical database model. A hierarchical database is a series of flat files, each one similar to a spreadsheet, that are linked in structured treelike relationships (see Fig. 11.2). Data are represented as a series of parent-child relationships. A patient's record (the parent) might link to "follow-up exam" children, and each of these children might link to the records of specialized procedures (grandchildren).

Each child segment can be linked to only one parent, and a child can only be reached through its parent. This could create a problem. The radiology department might want to have a patient's X ray results as its "children" whereas we would want to keep them with the appropriate set of follow-ups or perhaps store each exam as part of a master patient record. Will we need to make two or even three copies of the exam results?

To avoid data redundancy, all information in a hierarchical database is stored in a single location and referenced by links or physical pointers in other locations. For example, the "**patients**" record might contain actual data in the "specialized exam" segment, whereas the "**radiology**" record held only a pointer to the "specialized exam" data in "**patients**."

---

[33]The lack of an audit trail would meet with fatal objections from most regulatory agencies.

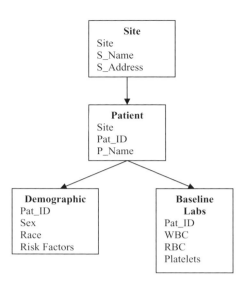

FIGURE 11.2 Hierarchical Database.

On the downside, the link established by the pointers is permanent and cannot be modified. A design originally optimized to work with the data in one way may prove totally inefficient in working with the data in other ways. The physical links make it very difficult to expand or modify the database; changes typically require substantial rewriting efforts and risk introducing errors and destroying irreplaceable data.

Network Database Model

The network database model (also known as CODASYL DBTG) provides for multiple paths among segments (that is, more than one parent-child relationship) (see Fig. 11.3). Unfortunately, with no restrictions on the number of relations, the database design can become overwhelmingly complex. Each new addition takes longer and longer to implement. Too often, changes that appear quick to implement at first take weeks to repair and implement correctly. The network model fails to provide the needed solution to our problems of storage and retrieval.

Relational Database Model

A relational database appears to stores all its data inside tables. Each table consists of a set of rows and columns similar (from the user's point of view, though not the computer's) to the rows and columns of

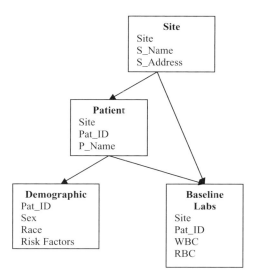

FIGURE 11.3 Network Database.

a spreadsheet. As with a spreadsheet, a row corresponds to a record and the columns to the data fields in the record.

Here's an example of a table and the SQL statement that creates the table:

Table: PAT_DEMOG				
Pat_ID	Sex	Brth_date	Race	Origin
071-1136	M	22/11/36	W	USA

```
CREATE TABLE Pat_Demog(
        PatID char (7),
        Sex char(1),
        Brth_date date,
                ....)
```

In a relational database, all operations on data are done on the tables themselves, although other tables may be produced as the result. You never see anything except for tables.

Two basic operations can be performed on a relational table. The first is retrieving a subset of the columns. The second is retrieving a subset of the rows. Here are samples of the two operations:

```
SELECT PatID, Sex FROM Pat_Demog
```

Pat_ID	Sex
001-421	M
002-043	M

```
SELECT * FROM Pat_Demog WHERE sex = "F"
```

Pat_ID	Sex	Brth_Date	Diabetes
002-044	F	26/12/37	No
002-047	F	08/08/54	No

The relational approach has several major advantages including:

- **Unlimited data access**
- **Easily modified data structure**
- **Ease of access**
- **Widely used query language**

Processing queries does not require predefined access paths among the data as in a network access database.

Changes to the database structure are easily accommodated. The structure of the database can be changed without having to change any applications that were based on that structure.

Here's an example: You add a new field for the patient's smoking habits in the patients' table. If you were using a nonrelational database, you would probably have to modify the application that will access this information by including "pointers" to the new data. With a relational database, the information is immediately accessible because it is automatically related to the other data by virtue of its position in the table. All that is required to access the new field is to add it to a SQL SELECT list.

Table: **Base_Lab**				
Pat_ID	Hemo	RBC	Platelets	WBC
001-421	43	5.01	205	5
001-424	13.4	4.28	248	11.9

The structural flexibility of a relational database allows combinations of data to be retrieved that were never anticipated at the time the database was designed. In contrast, the database structure in older database models is "hard-coded" into the application; if you add new fields to a nonrelational database, any applications that access the database will have to be updated.

The true power of the relational approach comes from the ability to operate simultaneously on several tables that do *not* have the same set of columns. Suppose you want to establish a relationship between the tables Pat_Demo and Base_LAB. These tables have a common column, the name of the company. Even if each table has its own name for the column, we see that the data stored and their meaning are the same on both tables. So we could use this relationship to get a URL for each person on ADDR_BOOK. Here's the SQL statement:

```
SELECT Pat_Dem.Sex, Base_Lab.WBC
   FROM Pat_Dem, Base_Lab
   WHERE Pat_Dem.Pat_ID = Base_Lab.Pat_ID.
```

This operation, matching rows from one table to another using one or more column value, is called a "join," more specifically an "inner join."

A final benefit not visualized by the inventors of the relational database is that SQL, the query language associated with System R, IBM's first attempt at a relational database, has become a standardized part of all relational software, so that regardless of what brand or version of relational database your company utilizes, the same set of commands will be used to extract information. This makes it easier to transfer or bring in new employees from outside your department.[34]

Which Database Model?

Both the network and hierarchical models make use of an Indexed Sequential Access Method, or ISAM to speed up data access and retrieval. Under ISAM, records are located by using a key value. A smaller index file stores the keys along with pointers to the records in the larger data file. The index file is first searched for the key, and then the associated pointer is used to locate the desired record.

If a database design is completely static (that is, the tables and columns do not change), then an ISAM-based application will typically provide faster retrieval times for 1) getting a single row by primary key; 2) getting a set of rows containing a particular

---

[34]Visit http://www.blnet.com/msqlpc to get links for more information about the SQL query language.

secondary key value; and 3) getting a row by key and processing all the rows that physically follow it in the database. Not surprisingly, many accounting systems today are based on the network or hierarchical model.

In contrast, the relational database excels at executing complex, ad hoc queries and lends itself to the management of clinical data.

Object-Oriented Databases

Object-oriented databases can work with images, spreadsheets, documents, CAD, e-mail messages, and directory structures, as well as text. From the computer's point of view, "data" is merely a sequence of bits (1's and 0's) residing in some sort of storage structure; perspective images are no more exotic than the characters that make up text. An object-oriented database could store ultrasound photos and ECG tracings alongside the numerical summary of results. Still, it is difficult to visualize the practical value this still-experimental approach could have for clinical trials. Let someone else be a pioneer.

CLIENTS AND SERVERS

Database management systems (DBMS), relational or otherwise, are heavily influenced by the processing architecture, that is, by how the work is divided between the host (usually a larger computer where the data is stored, a mainframe or a Unix-based minicomputer) and the client (your desktop PC or workstation). Older databases (like IMS) reside entirely on the host mainframe. All Microsoft Access data processing is done at the desktop. Somewhere in the middle is a client-server DBMS like Oracle.

I recommend the client-server approach. A database *server* is the component of a computer program that manages the database itself. The applications (queries) you and your staff work with are *clients* to the database server. In the client-server approach these applications never manipulate the database directly, but only make requests for the server to

---

WHO CHOOSES THE SOFTWARE?

Should your project be consistent with corporate guidelines? Although there is a great deal of value to having corporate guidelines for software purchases, including 1) reduced costs due to bulk purchase, 2) easier maintenance, and 3) ease of shifting programmers from department to department, one size seldom fits all. The key lies in knowing where to draw the boundaries.

Should clinical affairs be asked to use an inflexible decades-old data management system just because accounting does?

perform the operations. The server reduces the risk of data file corruption, because only the server writes to the database; a crash or power outage on a client desktop—a not infrequent occurrence—will not leave the database in an incomplete state.

A database server takes advantage of the client-server architecture to lower network usage. Here is how this works: If a client application were to open a file stored on a file server directly, it would need to retrieve and transfer every record across the network just to filter out the ones it really needs. Instead, the database server filters out the unneeded records and only sends out over the network the data that really matter. Microsoft's PC-based Access®is a relational database, but it is not a database server. MS-SQL, SQL Anywhere®, DB2®, and Oracle®are both relational databases and database servers.

One Size Does Not Fit All

Bumbling's Clinical Affairs Department insisted that all studies use not only the same data management system but the same database construction, the rationale being that this would further reduce development costs. Here's what actually happened:

- **The cost of developing the data analysis software doubled because of the constant need to extract and merge subsets before any analysis could be performed.**
- **Because so much of each file was waste space, devoted to variables not in the current study, retrieving the information proved enormously time consuming and almost brought the corporate mainframe to its knees.**
- **Information Systems kept buying larger and larger hard disks, but invariably ran out of space as the files with their hundreds of dummy variables were an order of magnitude larger than they should be.**
- **The complex keying instructions that resulted when several pieces of information had to be combined into one to "fit" the standard design introduced a large number of errors that had to be corrected.**
- **Programmers had to work overtime during the analysis phase designing programs that would unpack the data that had been combined and recoded during the keying process.**

COMBINING MULTIPLE DATABASES

For the reasons discussed in the preceding sections, we need to divide our data up among several files (or databases) and then find some

> **DOMAIN TABLES**
>
> Every time you have a column whose value must come from a known set of values you have a "domain" for that column. Your domain may be as simple as the day of the week (SUN, MON, TUE, . . . SAT), as lengthy as a list of anatomical sites, or partially unknown as the set of adverse events. Domain tables reduce storage requirements by associating an ID (or code) to a name or description. Whether the investigator enters a symptom name or its abbreviation, only one of the two (your choice) is permanently stored.
>
> In addition to providing the benefits of flexible data entry (accepting "close" misspellings such as "asperin"), domain tables provide faster queries, faster sorting, lower storage, and ease in updating. They're a standard part of most relational systems, present in both the least and the most expensive.

way of linking these files together. How should we divide the data up? A good rule of thumb is to combine all the information collected by a single individual at a single point of time in the same file.

We link the disparate files with the aid of keys. A *key* is an element of information common to several databases that serves to tie the databases together. One obvious key is the patient ID; another is the date on which a particular examination was completed.

The key item must be stored in each of the files it is to link. A patient's name is not a good choice for a key as it is something we wish to keep confidential and thus stored in as few locations as possible. A patient's sex, the length of a target lesion, or the dosage of the drug the patient is receiving are not good choices because their presence in more than one database would be redundant.

A good rule of thumb is to use the patient ID as a primary key to tie all the databases together and to use an examination date or some other value as a secondary key to tie together information that is closely related. An example of related data might be the adverse event form on which the need for a certain action was recorded along with all the databases containing the information related to that action.

A RECIPE FOR DISASTER

In Chapter 8, the importance of providing detailed instructions was illustrated with an example from an almost-successful study. The "almost" came about when Bumbling Pharmaceutical acquired the trial's sponsor shortly after the trials were under way. Severe errors in database construction (resulting from forcing the data to fit into the standard corporate data model) led to a subsequent failure to locate and recapture information essential to the analysis of treatment effects. Recovery was labor intensive and time consuming, resulting in substantial delays in completion of the study.

The company's first error lay in adopting an older hierarchical database management system in use by accounting. The rationale was that the product was already in use so the database programmers would not need to be retrained. Of course, these same programmers were already tied up with their work in accounting, so a whole new group had to be hired and trained in a system generally considered to be obsolete.

Bumbling's second and incurable error lay in setting up the database. Each of the case report forms was split into a half-dozen parts: investigator's signature and date to one file and the dates of various events to another. One whole file was reserved for keeping the dates of patients' visits. Unfortunately, there was no way (other than the dates themselves) to link these visits with the various follow-up forms.

An intricate coding system using a page name and an "event" would have worked had, for example, the one-month follow-up actually taken place exactly one month after the start of the intervention. But it never did, except on rare occasions.

If the occasional form did not get entered in the database (and because Bumbling was using paper forms for initial data entry, there were always forms that did not get entered in the database), one could never be sure which form went with which date in the visit register.

Although not explicitly stated in the original sponsor's protocol (as it ought to have been), good medical practice required that the taking of a repeat angiogram precede revascularization. The data indicating a repeat revascularization had been performed were (mainly) stored in one file whose possible keys included the patient's ID, an "event" ID, and the date of surgery. The data for the corresponding angiogram were stored in two separate files, neither of which contained the date on which the angiogram had been taken. The keys for these two files included the patient's ID, an "event" ID, and a "page" name.

A different coding system had been used for the event IDs than that used in the revascularization file, so it was impossible to reconcile the two.[35] Fortunately (?), there was a fourth file in which the dates of patient visits were often recorded; its possible keys included the patient ID, an "event" ID (using approximately the same coding system as the files), and the date of the visit. For revascularizations, the recorded visit date might or might not coincide with the date of surgery.

The only data that could be utilized for the automated (computer) analysis were results for which there was an unambiguous link between the angiogram and the revascularization. The angiograms for approximately 5% of the patients in the trial had simply fallen through the cracks.

Fortunately, after a lengthy inspection of the original records by hand, almost all were located. The programs used for analysis were modified to incorporate explicit reference to the individual patient records and to maintain a clear audit trail for the regulatory agency. The losses in money and time were absorbed in the company's profit and loss statement.

Bottom Line: Despite having a computer that could process a record every millisecond, the company ended up doing hand counts at a rate of one per minute. Kind of reminds you of the 2000 Florida Presidential election.

Transferring Data

Transferring the data entered at each physician's and each laboratory's computer to the central database can be done in one of three ways:

1. **Enter directly at each physician's computer.**
2. **Transfer the data automatically at day's end via telephone to the central database.**
3. **Copy the data each day to a CD; at the end of the week the CD is mailed to your staff to be entered into the database.**

Direct entry at each investigator's cite to the master database is ruled out because of the impossibility of maintaining a continuous link to multiple disparate computers that may be hundreds, even thousands of miles apart.

Which of the last two options to adopt will depend upon the volume of data you expect to receive from each treatment center.

---

[35]As with so many of Bumbling's efforts, no documentation was ever found for either coding system. Apparently, it had been left to each employee who quit, retired, or transferred to another department to brief his replacement.

With either alternative, a second data entry program "reads" the transmitted files and enters the records into the database. Human intervention is required only to start the program and slip the CD into the host computer's CD drive.

Separating the two stages of data entry guarantees that investigators' contact with the database is strictly limited. They can enter their data in the database, but they cannot modify it once it is entered. Nor can they access the database and be exposed to findings that might color their own observations.

Data Entry Via the Internet. A fourth alternative is to have the data collection forms stored on a single central computer to be accessed and completed via the Internet. The chief advantages of this approach are that updating and distribution of trial protocol and data collection forms can be accomplished at a single location so that fewer monitoring visits and monitoring personnel are required (See Lallas et al., 2004; Lopez-Carrero et al., 2005; Marks et al., 2001).

The offsetting disadvantages include:

- **High-speed Internet connections are required at each teminal.**
- **Real and perceived security threats may inhibit both patients and study centers from participating.**
- **The intervening Internet service providers as well as the Internet itself may be unavailable for varying periods.**
- **The industry is far from stable. Third-party Internet resources may cease to exist before the completion of the study.**

Note also that when data collection and verification is conducted via the Web, new data management methods and software may be required. See, for example, Brandt et al. (2000) and Wübbelt, Fernandez, and Heymer (2000).

QUALITY ASSURANCE AND SECURITY

Maintaining Patient Confidentiality

The patient's name, address and other identifying information should be stored in one file only, and access to that file should be severely restricted. References to patients in other files should be by coded ID only.

Access to Files

Although the ability to *write to and modify* a clinical database can and should be restricted to a privileged and responsible (and readily

> **STORE THE DATA YOU COLLECT**
>
> Although the date of discharge from the hospital was included on the case report forms, Bumbling Pharmaceuticals decided not to include this information in the database. The rationale for this deletion was lost after the database designer was promoted. Later, when it was realized the date of discharge was essential to a comparison of adverse events in the two treatment groups, the preliminary analysis had to be done by hand rather than by computer.
>
> To avoid bumbling yourself, always
> - Begin with your reports.
> - Plan for and collect the data you'll need for your reports.
> - Store the data you collect.
> - Store the data as they were entered.
> - Design the database in terms of one file or table for each set of data that was entered by the same person at the same point in time.

monitored) few, everyone with a need to know (CRMs, project leaders, project physicians) should be able to *access and read* from the database and, moreover, to do so in a manner no more difficult than the manner in which data are entered into it.

Your data management software should permit you to establish privileges on a file-by-file basis for every individual who will have access to the system. Too often, data managers and statistical analysts function as some kind of primitive priesthood, issuing proclamations that they and only they shall be privileged to access the clinical database. But with today's databases, security can be readily maintained while giving those with a need to know immediate access to the data they need.

A single individual, normally the database manager, is entrusted with issuing passwords and security levels to all those seeking access to the database.[36]

Full access would include the ability to read from, write to, update, and even delete files. These privileges are necessities while the database is still under construction. Full access after the database is constructed should be limited to the database manager and his assistants.

Access should be granted on a file-by-file basis. Access to the file containing a patient's name, address, and other identifying information and to the file containing the treatment assignments should be severely restricted. Read-only access to most of the other files should be made on a need-to-know basis. Here are two examples:

---

[36]Security levels are assigned both to individuals and to automated applications.

Name	Task	Read Baseline	Read Other	Write	Create	Copy
Art Wood	DBM	y	y	y	y	y
Brian Donleavy	Project Mgr	y	y			y
Jan Moore	CRM		y	y		y
Bill Woodson	CRM		y	y		
Mike Chuck	Statistician	y	y			
Seri Shanti	Programmer		y	y	y	

FIGURE 11.4 Tonto Project: Database Access Privileges.

1. The pathology laboratory should be able to both read and write to the file containing pathology reports.
2. Until the trials are complete, investigators should not be given direct access to the database, not even to their own data. Instead, they would submit a request to the CRM and the CRM would provide them with any needed data that is consistent with the guidelines you and your data manager have established.

While the database is under construction, the database manager normally makes all the decisions regarding who should have access to the database, the level of access they should have, and the files they should be permitted to access. Just before the start of full-scale data entry, the database manager should submit a chart similar to Figure 11.4 to you for your approval. Thereafter, all decisions as to access to the data will be yours alone.

Maintaining an Audit Trail

To avoid even the appearance of fraud, and to satisfy government regulations, all changes to the database must be automatically tracked and recorded by the system.

Security

The best approach to security is pure paranoia, although your chief concern is not theft but the integrity and safety of the database. Access by your competitors is seldom a problem. The very fact that you are conducting full-scale clinical trials tells them most of what they want to know. Other information they will attempt to glean from your employees.[37]

To protect the database, you will need to backup (copy) and test your data on a regular basis and store at least some of the backup

---

[37] The best solution to this latter problem is to ensure employee loyalty through ongoing effort. See Gandy (2001) and Mendes (1995).

copies in a remote location. Standard practice is the cycle of 3 (sometimes 5, and sometimes 7).

Backups are made on the evenings of days 1, 2, and 3. On the night of day 4, the backup of day 4 is sent to a remote location and the cycle is restarted; the backups of days 2 and 3 are discarded as days 5 and 6 backed up.

Although backing up the database and storing the backups at a remote location are essential, you'll need to do more. Backing up data that is already contaminated is pointless. You'll need to run tests on your database before a backup is made. These tests are particularly important during the early part of the trials when you are unlikely to be accessing the data on a regular basis.

Tests should be made on a file-by-file basis. Possible tests include:

- **Selecting five records at random from each file**
- **Counting the total number of records**
- **Printing out the minimum and maximum of at least two of the fields**

FOR FURTHER INFORMATION

Brandt CA; Nadkarni P; Marenco L; Karras BT; Lu C; Schacter L et al. (2000) Reengineering a database for clinical trials management: lessons for system architects. *Control Clin Trials* 21:440–461.

Date CJ. (1999) *An Introduction to Database Systems (Introduction to Database Systems)*, 7th ed. San Francisco: Addison-Wesley.

Garcia-Molina H; Ullman JD; Widom J. (1999) *Database System Implementation*. Upper Saddle River, NJ: Prentice Hall.

Gandy BG. (2001) *30 Days to a Happy Employee: How a Simple Program of Acknowledgment Can Build Trust and Loyalty at Work*. New York: Fireside.

Kelly MA; Oldham J. (1997) The Internet and randomised controlled trials. *Int J Med Inform* 47:91–99.

Lallas CD; Preminger GM; Pearle MS; Leveillee RJ; Lingeman JE; Schwope JP et al. (2004) Internet based multi-institutional clinical research: a convenient and secure option. *J Urol* 171:1880–1885.

Lopez-Carrero C; Arriaza E; Bolanos E; Ciudad A; Municio M; Ramos J; Hesen W. (2005) Internet in clinical research based on a pilot experience. *Contemp Clin Trials* 26:234–243.

Marks R; Bristol H; Conlon M; Pepine CJ. (2001) Enhancing clinical trials on the Internet. lessons from INVEST. *Clin Cardiol* 24:V17–V23.

Mendes A. (1995) *Inspiring Commitment: How to Win Employee Loyalty in Chaotic Times*. New York: McGraw-Hill Professional Publishing.

Paul J; Seib R; Prescott T. (2005) The Internet and clinical trials: background, online resources, examples and issues. *J Med Internet Res* 2005 7(1):e5.

Prokscha S. (1999) *Practical Guide to Clinical Data Management*. Englewood, CO: Interpharm.

Rondel RK; Varley SA; Webb C. (2000) *Clinical Data Management*, 2nd ed. New York: Wiley.

Wübbelt P; Fernandez G; Heymer J. (2000) Clinical trial management and remote data entry on the Internet based on XML case report forms. *Stud Health Technol Inform* 77:333–337.

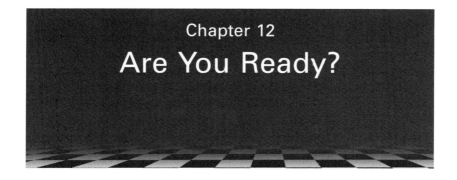

Chapter 12
Are You Ready?

THIS CHAPTER IS INTENDED to serve as a master checklist before you start the actual study. Hopefully, most of the points touched on here, many of them quite minor, have already been disposed of by your staff. But as with a vacation whose first few days are ruined because you forgot the mosquito repellent, a few extra moments of reflection before your departure can yield large dividends.

We begin by reviewing the basis of your study, the pharmaceuticals or devices that will be used in the intervention—you do have a full supply on hand?—and then go over points to be covered with your investigators and site coordinators, the final field tests of your questionnaires, data entry software and hardware, and uniform instructions to be issued to participants.

PHARMACEUTICALS/DEVICES

- **Preferably, all devices and drugs used in the study should be drawn from the same lot and set aside before the start of the study.** Obvious exceptions include prohibitively expensive devices that are normally manufactured on a just-in-time basis and pharmacological agents whose potency deteriorates quickly.
- **Controls should be matched to the active intervention on the basis of both appearance (size and color) and taste. The matching should be verified by your staff.**
- **All vials should be labeled with the patient's name, the patient's ID, and (if applicable) instructions for self-administration** (e.g., twice a day with meals).

A Manager's Guide to the Design and Conduct of Clinical Trials, by Phillip I. Good
Copyright ©2006 John Wiley & Sons, Inc.

- To monitor compliance, the patient should only be supplied with the amounts of pharmacological agents needed for use until the next scheduled checkup.
- The initial labeled supplies should have been shipped to the investigators.

SOFTWARE

- Data entry software is completely debugged and tested.
- The variables and layouts of the interim reports have been determined.
- Software for tracking recruitment is in place and has been tested.

HARDWARE

- All the computer hardware to be provided to investigators has been purchased and delivered.
- All units were equipped with software and tested in house before shipping to investigators.
- All units were installed and field tested at the individual investigators' sites.
- Service personnel whose primary responsibility is to maintain the equipment in the field have been hired and trained.

DOCUMENTATION

The following are complete and submitted or printed:

- Proposal
- Physician's manual
- Informed consent form
- Laboratory manuals
- Patient instructions

INVESTIGATORS

Investigators have been recruited. Your staff has visited the sites of all investigators and investigational laboratories. At each site you have done the following:

- Established the identity of the single individual who will be responsible for ensuring the orderly collection and monitoring of data.

- Conducted training programs for the chief investigator and all individuals who will have contact with patients or be involved in data entry.
- Provided copies of procedures manuals and of the forms to be given to patients. These latter include informed consent, study overview, and any instructions needed to ensure compliance.
- Supervised the installation of the data entry computer and field tested the software, the hardware, and the communication links with your office.

EXTERNAL LABORATORIES

Contracts, communication links, and protocols have been established with external laboratories.

REVIEW COMMITTEES

- Referral criteria determined. (Will the pathology committee review all biopsies or only those biopsies that are suspect or ambiguous?)
- Duties determined. (As an example, the safety committee will classify all adverse events as to whether or not they are treatment related.)
- Meeting arrangements determined. (For example, the members of the safety committee will each make an independent review, then teleconference monthly for a final determination.)
- All committee members recruited.

PATIENTS

- Recruitin g quotas determined for each treatment site.
- Recruiting methods determined subject to ongoing review.
- Patient instructions ready for field test.

REGULATORY AGENCY

- Agency has approved the trials.

TEST PHASE

In most case, it can be advantageous to hold a preliminary test phase at one or two sites to ensure that all systems are fully functional. The evaluation would include field tests and possible revision of

- **Drug/device delivery procedures**
- **Data entry software**
- **Transfer of data from the investigator to central storage**
- **Transfer of samples from investigator to external laboratory and of data from external laboratory to central storage**
- **Physician and laboratory manuals**
- **Recruitment procedures**
- **Patient instructions**

A report on these tests with a list of proposed modifications should be made to the implementation committee.

Chapter 13
Monitoring the Trials

AS WITH EACH OF THE MANY PROJECTS WITH which you as a manager will be associated, success can only be assured if you plan exhaustively (the focus of the last eight chapters), carefully monitor the project's progress (the topic of the next three chapters), and review the results to see what may be gained from your experiences for use in the future.

Ongoing monitoring is essential for all of the following:

- **Recruiting and retaining investigators**
- **Recruiting and retaining patients**
- **Protocol adherence**
- **Quality control**
- **Patient compliance**
- **Limiting adverse effects**

ROLES OF THE MONITORS

Most of the duties, if not all the responsibility, for monitoring the trials will fall upon the shoulders of the medical monitor and the clinical research monitors, or CRMs.

The medical monitor is responsible for

1. **Preliminary site visits at which the investigator's bona fides are established**
2. **Monitoring the progress of physician recruiting**
3. **Monitoring all remaining aspects of the trials including**
    a) Patient withdrawals and noncompliance
    b) Adverse events

A Manager's Guide to the Design and Conduct of Clinical Trials, by Phillip I. Good
Copyright ©2006 John Wiley & Sons, Inc.

c) Such other problems as are brought to her attention by the CRMs
4. Taking such corrective action as may be deemed appropriate including
   a) Arranging for review by an independent pathologist or radiologist
   b) Bringing protocol violations and excessive numbers of adverse events to the attention of internal and external review committees
5. Maintaining physician interest throughout lengthy trials

The medical monitor should write out the responsibilities of the clinical investigator, provide training in these responsibilities, remind investigators of their responsibilities as necessary, and with the assistance of the CRMs reward investigators for successful execution of their responsibilities.

The CRM is responsible for

- Preliminary visits to each site to ensure the smooth flow of data
- Monitoring the progress of patient recruiting
- Working with the statistician to develop interim reports and reviewing these reports on a regular basis
- Monitoring and correcting problems at the investigator's site including those related to
  - Drug/device delivery
  - Data entry
  - Transfer of data from the investigator to central storage
  - Procedures for treatment and observation
  - Availability of manuals and forms
- Maintaining physician interest throughout lengthy trials
- Follow-up site visits that serve both to maintain morale and to forestall problems with patients, the investigator, and the investigator's staff
- Picking up and verifying the signed, printed case report forms and seeing that the

CRM'S PRETRIAL CHECKLIST
Establish a delivery schedule for drugs/devices.
At each investigator's site ensure that
Initial supplies of drugs/devices are present.
Data entry hardware and software is installed and tested.
Training is completed.
Site coordinator is employed/appointed.
Informed consent forms are on hand.
Procedure manuals are on hand.
Instructions, containers, and labels for shipping to investigational laboratories are on hand.

> investigator is paid in timely fashion (I strongly recommend against separating the accounting function from that of the monitor.)
> - **Referring otherwise intractable problems to the medical monitor or project manager**

The level of monitoring will depend on the nature of the trial (Phase I, II, or III) and its intent. Monitors need to be aware of patient withdrawals and to discuss them either with the planning committee (if the withdrawals affect all sites) or with the specific investigators involved.

BEFORE THE TRIALS BEGIN

Before the trials begin your CRMs and medical monitor should already have met not once but several times with each investigator. The purpose of these meetings is threefold:

> 1. To survey the investigator's working arrangements
> 2. To establish rapport with and gain the trust of the investigator
> 3. To arrange for the appointment of a site coordinator

Establishing rapport is often quite difficult as the responsibilities borne by investigators tend to make them suspicious of all those without similar training. Physicians trust physicians; pilots trust pilots; and cops trust cops. Everyone else is a "civilian." Even the appointment of a site coordinator often meets with some resistance. Experienced monitors know that investigators tend to fall into one of three categories.

> 1. The "professional" understands both the need for and the value of a site coordinator and is eager to turn over the responsibilities.
> 2. The "do-it-myselfer" actively resists the appointment.
> 3. The "amateur" appears to go along with the request but actually sabotages it, appointing a temporary employee or a nurse who is about to depart on maternity leave.

Each category requires quite different treatment.

The experienced monitor understands the value of the professional and does not impose upon her time. Direct contacts with the professional—phone calls and visits—are kept to a minimum. Only when there are problems that cannot be resolved by the site coordinator is direct contact made.

The professional should be provided with regular progress reports concerning the study as a whole. "Rewards" could take the form of tickets to some event in which the investigator has expressed an interest.

The "do-it-myselfer" requires additional reassurance before being willing to delegate authority. She should be reminded that invariably she will be called away at a critical moment and, in any event, will need to designate a subordinate to take over her duties when she is summoned to an investigator's meeting. (You needn't actually have scheduled an investigator's meeting to utilize this ploy.)

If all else fails, the monitor should simply say that company policy requires that a site coordinator be appointed.

The project manager and medical monitor must back up the CRM on this point. It is essential to the validity of the study that the CRM meet with every member of the investigator's staff who will have any contact with patients in the study. Absent such contact, the investigator cannot be allowed to participate.

Monitors should make frequent contact with this type of investigator both before and during the study. To forestall problems, an experienced CRM makes it a point to notify the investigator before any contact with the site coordinator. This type of investigator should be provided with frequent progress reports on the conduct of the study.

The "amateur" also requires extended contact until the need for a full-time study coordinator working under the authority of the investigator is understood. One possible motive for a lack of cooperation is the need of the investigator to retain her staff for other purposes. Be prepared to either pay for an on-site coordinator or forgo the investigator's services. This type of investigator also requires frequent monitoring initially.

KICK-OFF MEETINGS

It is almost a tradition in the pharmaceutical industry that each set of clinical trials shall be preceded by a kick-off meeting at which the investigators are wined and dined at some exclusive retreat. We see no value in this. Indeed, such meetings often have a negative impact, with various groups of investigators reaching independent informal agreements on how they will conduct their portion of the study.

It is far better to reserve discretionary funds for morale-building meetings midway through or near the close of multiyear trials. Such follow-up meetings can also be used to go over aspects of the trials that have shown wide divergence among investigators.

TABLE 13.1 Monitoring Responsibilities

QC Function	Responsible Party
Protocol development, patient brochure development	The manager of trial design and development has primary responsibility assisted by full design team. The project manager and medical affairs will review them.
Drug/device quality and delivery	Manufacturing
CRF and CRF completion instructions	Project manager, software manager, and data manager. Cross-functional review and approval by biostatistics, CRMs, and medical affairs.
Instruction manuals	Design team, medical manager, and medical writing perform initial review. Followed by CRM and user acceptance testing.
Database design, data storage	Before release: • Peer review by programmers, testing, data manager • User acceptance testing (entry of mock data, comparison of input vs. output) Ongoing: data manager; QC programmer Locked for a report: QC programmer with review by data manager and statistician.
Site readiness and compliance (eligibility, informed consent, Rx regimen, follow-up, and GCPs)	CRMs and project manager
Protocol deviation identification and corrective action	CRMs, medical manager, with assistance from biostatistics, QC programmer.
Statistical analysis and report preparation	Biostatistics, medical monitor, lead investigators, project manager, and medical editor

DUTIES DURING TRIAL

Physician liaison is easily a full-time job. (If a study takes five years, the full-time job will last all five.) Most common problems can be solved by effective communication between the monitors and the investigator.

The efforts of the monitors may need to be supplemented by those of programmers, document writers, field engineers, the statistician, and virtually anyone who participated in the development phase.

Site Visits

Site visits need to be disciplined and organized, with the organization taking place before the monitor leaves his or her office. This includes reviewing all previously submitted forms to see whether they have been completed unambiguously. (See also under the heading "quality control" in Chapter 14.) Too frequent use of "other" and "unspecified" categories should be a red flag. The frequencies of adverse events, missing forms, and patient withdrawal should be compared with those at other study sites.

I recommend that each visit include a sit-down meeting with the investigator and/or the site coordinator whether or not there are problems. The purpose of such a meeting is primarily motivational, to share with the investigator information concerning the overall status of the project. Of ongoing concern is the priority the investigator is giving to your clinical trial—it cannot be allowed to drop off his or her viewing screen. Additional compensation should be provided (tickets to movies or sports events or a restaurant gift coupon) on an ongoing basis to the individual(s) responsible for data entry at each site.

Visits should rarely be made on a fixed frequency to a given location. A site should be visited more frequently and the stay be of longer duration if the site is new to the study or has a prior history of problems.

At least one visit should be made simply to ensure

- **Assignment to treatment is adhered to—in inadequately monitored single-blind studies, physicians have been known to ignore the treatment assignment from day 1.**
- **Treatment procedures are adhered to.**
- **Data recording methods are adhered to.**
- **Informed consent forms are administered correctly.**
- **Samples and specimens requiring off-site review are being dispatched promptly.**

Sites with novice investigators, lagging enrollment, delays in submission of informed consent and other forms, and or exceptional frequencies of adverse events should be visited more frequently.

The project manager needs to oversee the monitors' schedules; personality conflicts are not unknown, and there is a natural reluctance on anyone's part to return to an area where a hostile reception is anticipated.

Between Visits

The CRMs should remain in contact with investigators and supporting laboratories between visits so as to be aware of any or all of the following:

1. **Staff turnover**
2. **Changes in investigator's other responsibilities**
3. **Changes in facilities**
4. **Patient deaths or severe adverse reactions**

5. Protocol deviations
6. Cost overruns
7. Loss of interest

Staff Turnover. In the event of excessive staff turnover, be prepared to provide supporting staff and to train new personnel.

Changes in Responsibilities. One reason for remaining in ongoing contact with investigators and their staff is try to head off diversions of the investigator's time. In the event, you may have to monitor the investigator's activities more closely and revise downward your estimate of the number of patients likely to be treated at that site.

Changes in Facilities. Changes in facilities range from construction that forces patients to wait in the hall to out-of-alignment measuring devices to data entry terminals that have been unplugged. Working together, the CRM and the site coordinator can often resolve many of the resulting problems.

For example, although screaming at a hospital administrator will not generate more space in an already crowded institution, direct contact with study subjects who have been inconvenienced can be used to motivate them to remain with the study.

Occasionally, a monitor is confronted with a series of handwritten data entry forms and is told that the computer has been down for a week or two. Too late to ask, "Why wasn't I informed?" The solution lies with training, with encouraging the investigator's staff to contact your staff if there are further problems, and, not least, with following through on such contacts.

Patient Deaths or Severe Reactions. In the event of patient deaths or severe reactions, the investigator will often want to crack the treatment code. She should be discouraged from doing so until the medical monitor has had the opportunity for a thorough review of the case.

Deviations from Protocol. Deviations from protocol including modification of treatment without notification cannot be allowed to go undetected or unremarked. Immediate face-to-face contact by the medical monitor with the offending investigator is called for. Listening is always more effective than telling, but, inevitably, agreement to future adherence must be reached or the investigator's services terminated.

Loss of Interest. Loss of interest is not infrequent in long-term studies. We consider a variety of methods for handling the problem in the following section of this chapter. I strongly urge the production and distribution of a newsletter reporting on the trials at between two- and three-month intervals as an inexpensive method for both maintaining interest and disseminating information.

Cost Overruns. Depending on the type of billing arrangements, either you or the investigator may first realize that expenses at the investigator's site are excessive. The CRM's responsibility is to document all the expenses involved and be in a position to compare them with expenses at other sites. If it is the investigator who feels aggrieved, the CRM (and the medical monitor) must listen and respond to the investigator's feelings.

The possible actions you as project manager might take are discussed under budgeting in Chapter 14. Because of the monitors' continuing need to maintain rapport with investigators, I would recommend a third party be the one dispatched to work with the investigator if corrective action is called for.

NEVER GIVE AN ADVANCE, OR HOW 300 PATIENTS TURNED INTO 75

Several years ago I was called in as a consultant by a medical device firm, ostensibly to do a survival analysis requested by a federal agency, but in actuality (the almost invariable case when a consultant is brought in) to be the bearer of bad news concerning the many failed aspects of the study.

The data management system crashed regularly. The database was filled with discrepancies, and there were no procedures in place for remedying them. As I proceeded step by step with the analysis, the 300 case report forms that had been filed so promisingly at the beginning of the study were reduced to 75 when I looked at the follow-ups. Five of the missing forms could be found on the CRM's desk—the rest simply had never been submitted (and, in some instances, never completed) by the physician.

You'd think the cardiologists would have wanted their money. They'd done the work; all they had to do was return the forms and the dollars would follow.

"They've already been paid," was the unexpected response. "Most are friends of the president of our company, he's a physician, too, and he made sure they were paid promptly."

Without checking to see if they'd done the work?

"Without checking."

As it turns out, this company's device did increase the survival rate of the cardiac patients who were fortunate enough to receive it. But it took the company another year before sufficient data were on hand to validate their claim and another year of deferred profits (and wasted lives) before their product could be brought to market.

Other Duties

Other duties of the monitors during the trials include

- **Arranging for payment of physicians and testing laboratories as completed reports are received (see sidebar)**
- **Monitoring adverse effects, a topic we consider at length in Chapter 14**
- **Revising interim reports**
- **Maintaining physician interest in lengthy trials**

Although sketches of the form and layout of the interim reports will have been developed before the trials, details invariably will evolve during the trials. For example, frequencies may be replaced or supplemented by percentages, graphs supplement text, and additional breakdowns by patient and disease characteristics required. The CRM and medical monitor may also need to request comprehensive workups for specific sites that the monitor intends to visit.

MAINTAINING PHYSICIAN INTEREST IN LENGTHY TRIALS

With patients being recruited into the study over a long period of time, participating physicians may lose interest when they fail to see dramatic results in patients who are further along in the process. Look to physician motivations to ensure retention. Often what was a motivating factor at the start of the trials proves less rewarding than hoped for or even turns into an irritant.

Let's take a second look at the list of potential motivators that was provided in the chapter on physician recruiting:

1. Enhance one's career—but only if the trial is paying off.
2. Participate in scientifically exciting research—if familiarity breeds contempt, a refresher course is called for.
3. Obtain medical benefits for one's patients—again, you may need to remind the physician of the nature of these benefits; a brief irregular newsletter, distributed in both hard copy and e-mail form can prove valuable.
4. Obtain new medical or scientific equipment provided by sponsors to enable trial (or purchased with monies only available downstream)—if already purchased the investigator may have come to view such equipment as his own; three or four months into the trials would be the ideal time to affix a plaque to each piece of donated equipment.
5. Publish scientifically and medically important article—again, this is only a motivator if it appears there will be positive publishable results.

6. Obtain new staff to help with clinical trial—may come to be viewed as a burden as the physician begins to think of the staff as her own; summoning all such staff to your offices for a one-day meeting can provide an essential reminder.

Some motivators remain of continued importance, providing investigators do not forget who their source is:

7. Obtain money that may be used for personal interests.
8. Obtain money that may be used to conduct unsponsored trails of professional interest.
9. Enhance one's standing in an academic department because of bringing in grant money.
10. Develop a long-term relationship with a sponsor.
11. Repay a favor (can only be pushed so far).

With these latter motivators, you may need to adopt a carrot and stick approach, withholding monies or offering additional inducements. As always, the most cost-effective approach is to make the investigator feel part of a larger, inherently rewarding group experience.

Chapter 14
Managing the Trials

IN CHAPTER 14 WE CONSIDERED those activities for which the CRM and medical monitor bear primary responsibility. In this chapter we consider those functions where the CRM's role is secondary, though equally essential, as a highly skilled triage coordinator and data gatherer.

The day may come when some advanced AI-equipped cyborg will take over the CRM's monitoring activities; until then, we must rely on humans to go over the interim reports and take whatever actions are warranted.

Examining a report on recruitment, for example, the CRM must determine whether the problem can be localized to a few sites or is more widespread. She must decide whether the site merely requires moral encouragement or whether more active intervention is warranted. Should the medical monitor be notified and requested to intervene? Or can the CRM handle the problem alone?

Similarly, the CRM must decide whether to take direct action in problems involving withdrawals, missing data, or requests from investigators for additional information or guidance, or to refer the problems and requests to other individuals.

Problems may arise with any or all of the following

- **Recruitment**
- **Supplies of devices/drugs/biologics, sample collection kits, forms**
- **Late and incomplete forms**
- **Dropouts and withdrawals**
- **Protocol violations**
- **Adverse events**

A Manager's Guide to the Design and Conduct of Clinical Trials, by Phillip I. Good
Copyright ©2006 John Wiley & Sons, Inc.

You cannot collect too much information about trial progress. Some check points are obvious—for example, the number of follow-up forms in hand—until you ask where the lab results associated with those follow-upsare. The solution in this specific case is to track samples both as they reach the laboratory and as the results are entered into your database.

RECRUITMENT

The statistician can play an invaluable role in this function by developing forecasting models for recruitment. In those instances where recruitment is essentially passive—with prospective subjects appearing at investigators' offices purely as a matter of chance—forecasting is relatively straightforward. In Figure 14.1a, a simple linear regression model provides an appropriate forecast.

The response to active recruiting tends to take the form shown in Figure 14.1b of a sharp rise followed by a relatively slow drop-off in numbers. If a second recruiting campaign is launched a short time later as in Figure 14.1c, it tends to have a similar form, although with the numbers recruited being appreciably smaller than before. The trick to forecasting is realizing when the point of diminishing returns is reached and further investment in recruiting would be a waste of time.

Note: Haidich and Ioannidis (2003) find that sites (and physicians) that start late seldom make a useful contribution. Better to look elsewhere for new recruits.

SUPPLIES

What value can there be in recruiting a patient if the treating physician is not in possession of the appropriate informed consent forms, drugs (or devices or biologics), or sample collection kits. Presumably, it is the CRM who will track shortages. But who at the trial center will be responsible for making up deficiencies? How can delays be avoided or minimized? Obviously, a link needs to be maintained between the project manager and production and supplies on hand continually matched to forecast needs.

LATE AND INCOMPLETE FORMS

Late and incomplete forms are the major source of cost overruns and trial delays. They cannot be tolerated. Automated transfer of data

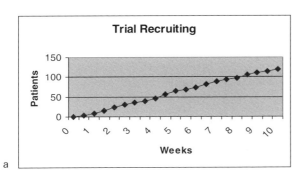

a

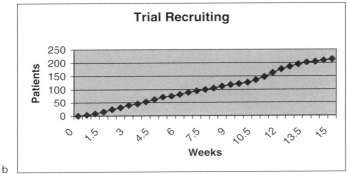

b

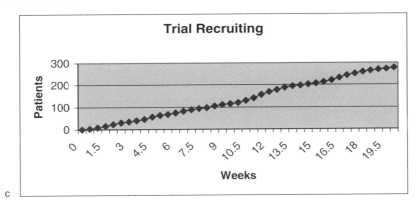

c

FIGURE 14.1

simplifies the preparation of a summary report detailing the forms received and the date of the next form due by site and patient ID. This report should be updated and reviewed daily by the CRM. Overdue and incomplete forms should be flagged as in Table 14.1.

The standard procedure for dealing with delays is as follows:

TABLE 14.1 CRFs from Examining Physician—Oct 10, 1999

Site	Patient	Elig	Baseline	2 wk	1 mo	2 mo	3 mo	6 mo	1 yr
001	100	6/3/99	6/18/99	7/8/99	7/22/99	8/25/99	**9/25/99**		
001	101	7/8/99	8/01/99	8/15/99	8/31/99	9/30/99	10/30/99		

1. The CRM places a telephone call to the site coordinator to determine the source of the difficulty.
2. She does what she can to facilitate collection and transmission of the needed information.
3. If the missing data involve several patients at the same site, she may choose to visit the site or to refer the matter to the medical monitor.
4. In turn, the medical monitor may either deal with the problem(s) or refer them to the project manager.
5. The primary responsibility of the project manager is to ensure that procedures are in place and that decisions are made not deferred.

DROPOUTS AND WITHDRAWALS

Missing or delayed forms are your first indication of problems involving dropouts or withdrawals. The first step is to determine whether the problem can be localized to one or two sites. If the problems are widespread, they should be referred to the biostatistician (who has access to the treatment code) to determine whether the withdrawals are treatment related.

Problems that can be localized to a few sites are best dealt with by a visit to that site. Widespread problems should be referred to an internal committee to determine the action to be taken.

> **CLINICAL TRIALS REPRESENT A LONG-TERM COMMITMENT**
>
> Bumbling lost interest in their Brethren device test midway through when they realized the results just weren't going to come out the way they planned. They probably would have shelved the project indefinitely had not it been brought forcefully to their attention that when you experiment with human subjects, the government insists on knowing the results whether or not they favor your product.

PROTOCOL VIOLATIONS

Suspected protocol violations should be referred to the medical monitor for immediate follow-up action.

As discussed in Chapter 7, a variety of corrective actions are possible, from revising the procedures manual if its ambiguity is the source of the problem to severing ties with a recalcitrant investigator. The CRM is responsible for recording the action taken and continues to be responsible for monitoring the out-of-compliance site.

ADVERSE EVENTS

Excessive numbers of serious adverse events can result in decisions to modify, terminate, or extend trials in progress.

Comments from investigators along with ongoing monitoring of events will provide the first indications of potential trouble.

Comments from investigators commonly concern either observed "cures" (generally acute) or unexpected increases in adverse events. Both are often attributed by investigators to the experimental treatment, even though in a double-blind study the code has not yet been broken.

As far as isolated incidents are concerned, Ayala and MacKillop (2001) question whether the treatment ever need be revealed to obtain improved care for the patient. Berger (2005) discusses the consequences of such revelations on the trials as a whole.

At the first stage of a review, the CRM, perhaps working in conjunction with the medical monitor, compares the actual numbers with the expected frequency of events in the control or standard group. If the increase appears to be of clinical significance, the statistician is asked to provide a further breakdown by treatment code.

Although the statistician will report the overall results of her analysis, neither the CRM nor the medical monitor who work directly with the investigators should come in direct contact with the uncoded data. For the same reason, only aggregate and not site-by-site results should be reported.

If the results of the analysis are not significant or of only marginal statistical significance (at, say, the 5% level), the trials should be allowed to continue uninterrupted.

If the results are highly significant, suggesting either that the new treatment has a distinct advantage over the old, or that it is inherently dangerous, a meeting of the external review committee should be called.

QUALITY CONTROL

Quality control is an ongoing process. It begins with the development of unambiguous questionnaires and procedure manuals and ends only with a final analysis of the collected data. Whether or not a CRO has been employed for forms design, database construction, data collection, or data analysis, the sponsor of the trials must establish and maintain its own program of quality control.

Interim quality control has four aspects:

1. Ensuring the protocol is adhered to, a topic discussed in chapter 13
2. Detecting discrepancies between the printed or written record and what was recorded in the database, a problem minimized by the use of electronic data capture
3. Detecting erroneous or suspect observations
4. Putting procedures in place to improve future quality

The use of computer-assisted direct data entry has eliminated most discrepancies of the first type, with the possible exceptions of the results of specialty laboratories that are used so infrequently that supplying them with computers would not have been cost effective and the findings of external committees that are normally provided in letter form.

Confirmation and validation of specialty laboratory results is normally done in person, perhaps no more often than once every three months.

The findings of external committees often arrive well after the other results are in hand. They are often transcribed and kept in spreadsheet form. Although such spreadsheets can be used as a basis for analysis, I'd recommend that they be entered into the database as soon as possible. Here's why: The spreadsheet often is too convenient, with the result that multiple copies are soon made, each copy differing subtly from the next with none ever really being the master. A single location for the data makes it easier to validate each and every record against the original printed findings of the external committee.

The project manager has the responsibility of making personnel assignments that will cover *all* aspects of quality. This translates to the creation and maintenance of a second team. For example, the individual responsible for verifying the entries on a specific data collection form cannot be among those who designed the form or created the database in which the form is stored.

VISUALIZE THE DATA

Recall our discussion in Chapter 2 of the sick monkey the United States spent millions puttig into orbit. Alan Hochberg, Vice President for Research at the ProSanos Corporation, reminds us that it is essential to visualize our data. "Discrepancies seldom leap out at you from a table."

One quick way to detect suspect observations, particularly for calculated fields, is to prepare a frequency diagram. In Figure 14.2,

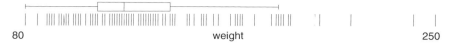

FIGURE 14.2 Display of Weights of 187 Young Adolescent Female Patients with a Box and Whiskers Plot Superimposed Above. The two largest values of 241 and 250 pounds seem suspicious. Better double check the case report forms.

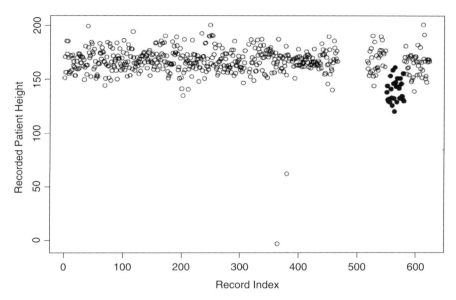

FIGURE 14.3 Detecting Data Entry Errors Through Data Visualization. Figure provided by Alan Hochberg and Ronald Pearson, ProSanos Corporation.

prepared with Stata©, a set of ultrahigh observations well separated from the main curve stands out from the rest. Sorting the data quickly reveals the source of the suspect values; the SAS Univariate procedure, for example, automatically tabulates and displays the three largest and smallest values.

Figure 14.3 provides a second example of how erroneous data entry may be detected through data visualization. The plotted data represent patient heights recorded in a multicenter clinical study. The data are grouped horizontally on a center-by-center basis. Note the blank space, representing missing data from one center. The solid dots represent data from a particular site, where the average patient was 10 inches shorter than elsewhere. An age histogram ruled out a predominance of pediatric or elderly patients as a cause of this

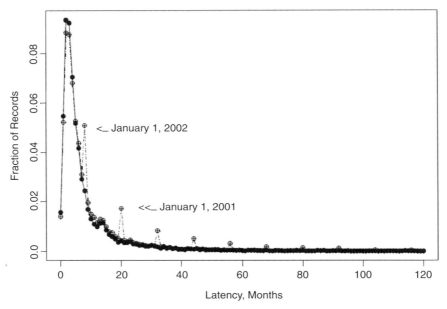

FIGURE 14.4 Using Data Visualization to Uncover Disguised Missing Data. Latency times represent the interval between the actual adverse event and the end of the calendar quarter in which is was included in an AERS data release. Figure provided by Alan Hochberg and Ronald Pearson, ProSanos Corporation.

anomaly, which was eventually tracked to incorrect coding: Patient heights of 5'1" were coded as "51 inches", 5'3" as "53 inches", etc. This anomaly was not detected by standard "edit checks" on ranges, because each individual data point was valid, and only the aggregate was anomalous.

Figure 14.4 shows us how disguised missing data may be recognized through data visualization. This histogram appeared during an evaluation of the promptness of reporting in the FDA Adverse Event Reporting System (AERS). The latency times plotted represent the interval between the actual adverse event and the end of the calendar quarter in which it was included in an AERS data release. The sharp periodic peaks represent dates that were coded as "January 1," rather than as "Missing," even though a missing data coding option is provided for in the AERS database. This is a case of "disguised missing data." Data on a finer scale show definite but smaller anomalous peaks on the first of each month.

Figure 14.5 shows how center-to-center variability in patient mix may be detected through data visualization. Although the mean

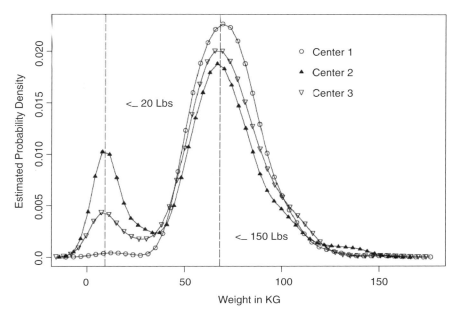

FIGURE 14.5 Figure provided by Alan Hochberg and Ronald Pearson, ProSanos Corporation. Density estimates were calculated using S-PLUS® (Insightful Corp., Seattle, WA).

weights at three centers are similar, the distributions differ substantially, reflecting substantial differences among the pediatric populations at each institution.

ROLES OF THE COMMITTEES

Recall that external committees serve three main functions:

1. **Interpretation of measurements—Does the ECG reveal an irregular heartbeat?**
2. **Assigning causes for adverse events—Was the heart attack related to treatment?**
3. **Advising on all decisions related to modifying, terminating, or extending trials in progress**

We consider the functions of the first two types of committee in this section and of the latter trial review and safety committee in the following section.

The initial meeting of each committee should be called by the medical monitor. Procedures for resolving conflicts among committee members (rule by majority or rule by consensus with secondary and tertiary review until consensus is reached) should be established.

After the initial meeting, members of these committees no longer need, in theory, to meet face to face. At issue is whether decisions should be made independently in the privacy of their offices or at group sessions. This problem is an organizational one. Will less time be spent in contacting members one by one (the tardy as well as the prompt) to determine their findings? Or in delaying meeting until a group session can be scheduled?

The chief problems related to these committees have to do with the dissemination of observations to committee members, the collection of results, and the entry of results into the computer.

Today, digital dissemination on a member-by-member basis is to be preferred to the traditional group meeting. Problems will arise only if a committee member lacks a receiving apparatus. It is common to use the same individuals on multiple studies, thus justifying the purchase of such equipment for them.

Members should be given a date for return of their analysis. The CRM should maintain a log of these dates, following up with immediate reminders should a date pass without receipt of the required information.

The CRM should maintain a spreadsheet on which to record findings from committee members as they are received. Spreadsheet data may then be easily entered into the database by direct electronic conversion.

Committee members require the same sort of procedure manuals and the same sort of follow-ups as investigators.

TERMINATION AND EXTENSION

Several stages and many individuals are involved in decisions to modify, terminate, or extend trials in progress. In this section, we detail the procedures and decisions involved.

A meeting of the external safety review committee should be called if either there have been an excessive number of adverse events or a medically significant difference between treatments has become evident.

The statistician should prepare a complete workup of all the findings as she would for a final report. The medical monitor should convey the findings to the external review committee. The CRMs and the statistician should accompany him in case the committee has questions for them.

The safety committee has two options:

1. **To recommend termination of the trials because of the adverse effects of the new treatment**
2. **To recommend modification of the trials**

Such modification normally takes the form of an unbalanced design in which a greater proportion of individuals are randomized to the more favorable treatment. See, for example, Armitage (1985), Lachin et al. (1988), Wei et al. (1990), and Ivanaova and Rosenberger (2000). Li, Shih, and Wang (2005) describe a two-stage design.

In such an *adaptive design*, the overall risk to the patients is reduced without compromising the integrity of the trials. The only "cost" is several more days of the statistician's time and several minutes of the computer's.

At issue in some instances is whether individuals who are already receiving treatment should be reassigned to the alternative treatment. Any such decision would have to be made with the approval of the regulatory agency.

A WORD OF CAUTION OF SPECIAL INTEREST TO CUBS FANS

Although tempting, decoded results, broken down by treatment, should *not* be monitored on a continuous basis. As any stock broker or any Cubs fan will tell you, short-term results are no guarantee of long-term success.

In July of 2001, baseball's Chicago Cubs were in the lead once again, a full six games ahead of their nearest interdivision opponent. Sammy Sosa, their right fielder, seemed set to break new records.[38] Moreover, the Cubs had just succeeded in acquiring one of Major League Baseball's most reliable hitters. Success seemed guaranteed.

Considering that the last time the Cubs won the overall baseball championship was in 1906, a twenty-game lead might have been better. The Cubs completed the 2001 season completely out of the running.

Statistical significance early in clinical trials when results depends on only a small number of patients offers no guarantee that the final result will be statistically significant as well. A series of such statistical tests taken a month or so apart is no more reliable. In fact, when repeated tests are made using the same data, the standard single-test p-values are no longer meaningful.

Sequential tests, where the decisions whether to stop or continue are made on a periodic basis, are possible but require quite complex statistical methods for their interpretation. See, for example, Slud and Wei (1982), DeMets and Lan (1984), Siegmund (1985), and Mehta et al. (1994).

---

[38]He later broke several.

In any event, observations on individuals already enrolled should continue to be made until the original date set for termination of the follow-up period. This is because a major purpose of virtually all clinical trials is to investigate the degree of chronic toxicity, if any, that accompanies a novel therapy. For this reason, among others, notably absent from our list of alternatives is the decision to terminate the trials at an early stage because of the demonstrable improvement provided by the new treatment.

EXTENDING THE TRIALS

After a predetermined number of individuals have completed treatment, but before enrollment ceases, the project manager should authorize the breaking of the code by the statistician and the completion of a preliminary final analysis.

As previously noted, the statistician should be the only one with access to the decoded data and results should be reported on an aggregate, not a site-by-site, basis.

If significant differences among treatment groups are observed, then the results may be submitted to an external committee for review. If the original termination date is only a few weeks away, then the trials should be allowed to proceed to completion.

If the differences among treatments are only of borderline significance, the question arises as to whether the trials should be extended in order to reach a definitive conclusion. Weighing in favor of such a decision would be if several end points rather than just one point in the desired direction.[39] Again the matter should be referred to the external committee for a decision, and if an extension is favored by the committee, permission to extend the trials should be requested from the regulatory agency.

BUDGETS AND EXPENDITURES

I cannot stress sufficiently the importance of keeping a budget and making an accounting of all costs incurred during the project. This information will prove essential when you begin to plan for future endeavors.

Obvious expenditures include fees to investigators, travel monies, and the cost of computer hardware and over-the-counter software.

---

[39] A multivariate statistical analysis may be appropriate; see Pesarin (2001).

Time is an expenditure. Because most of us, yourself included, will be working on multiple projects during the trials, a timesheet should be required of each employee and a group of project numbers assigned to each project.

Relate the work hours invested to each phase of the project. Track the small stuff including time spent on the telephone. The time recorded can exceed 8 hours a day and 40 hours a week and often does during critical phases of a clinical trial. (These worksheets also provide a basis for arguing that additional personnel are required.)

A category called "waiting-for" is essential. With luck—see Chapter 16—we can avoid these delays the next time around. Also of particular importance in tracking are tasks that require time-consuming manual intervention such as reconciling entries in "other" classifications and clarifying ambiguous instructions.

Midway through the project, you should be in a position to finalize the budget. Major fixed costs will already have been allocated and the average cost per patient determined.

If you've followed the advice given here, then even the programming required for the final analysis should be 99% complete—and so too will be the time required for the analysis. Although developing programs for statistical analysis is a matter of days or weeks, executing the completed programs against an updated or final database takes only a few minutes. Interpretation may take a man-week or more with several additional man-weeks for the preparation of reports.

Ours is a front-loaded solution. Savings over past projects should begin to be realized at the point of three-quarters completion, with the comparative numbers looking better and better with each passing day.

If you've only just adopted the use of electronic data capture, there may or may not be a record of past projects against which the savings can be assessed. The costs of "rescue efforts" often get buried or are simply not recorded. Thus the true extent of your savings may never be known. All the more reason for adopting the Plan-Do-Check approach in your future endeavors. Undoubtedly, changes in technology will yield further savings.

FOR FURTHER INFORMATION
Armitage P. (1985) The search for optimality in clinical trials. *Int Stat Rev* 53:15–24.

Artinian NT; Froelicher ES; Vander Wal JS. (2004) Data and safety monitoring during randomized controlled trials of nursing interventions. *Nurs Res* 53:414–418.

Ayala E; MacKillop N. (2001) When to break the blind. *Applied Clin Trials* 10:61–62.

Berger VW. (2005) *Selection Bias and Covariate Imbalances in Randomized Clinical Trials.* Chichester: John Wiley & Sons.

DeMets DL; Lan G. (1984) An overview of sequential methods and their application in clinical trials. *Commun Stat Theory Meth* 13:2315–2338.

Fleming T; DeMets DL. (1993) Monitoring of clinical trials: issues and recommendations. *Control Clin Trials* 14:183–197.

Gillum RF; Barsky AJ. (1974) Diagnosis and management of patient noncompliance. *JAMA* 228:1563–1567.

Haidich AB; Ioannidis JP. (2003) Late-starter sites in randomized controlled trials. *J Clin Epidemiol* 56:408–415.

Hamrell MR, ed. (2000) *The Clinical Audit In Pharmaceutical Development.* New York: Marcel Dekker.

Ivanova A; Rosenberger WF. (2000) A comparison of urn designs for randomized clinical trials of K > 2 treatments. *J Biopharm Stat* 10:93–107.

Lachin JM; Matts JP; Wei LJ. (1988) Randomization in clinical trials: conclusions and recommendations. *Control Clin Trials* 9:365–374.

Li G; Shih WJ; Wang Y. (2005) Two-stage adaptive design for clinical trials with survival data. *J Biopharm Stat* 15:707–718.

Mehta CR; Patel NR; Senchaudhuri P; Tsiatis AA. (1994) Exact permutational tests for group sequential clinical trials. *Biometrics* 50:1042–1053.

Pesarin F. (2001) *Multivariate Permutation Tests: With Applications in Biostatistics.* New York: Wiley.

Siegmund H. (1985) *Sequential Analysis: Tests and Confidence Intervals.* New York; Springer.

Slud E; Wei LJ. (1982) Two-sample repeated significance tests based on the modified Wilcoxon statistic. *JASA* 77:862–868.

Wei LJ; Smythe RT; Lin DY; Park TS. (1990) Statistical inference with data-dependent treatment allocation rules. *JASA* 85:156–162.

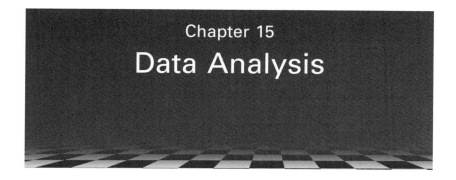

Chapter 15
Data Analysis

IN THIS CHAPTER WE REVIEW THE TOPICS you'll need to cover in your analysis of the data and the differing types of data you will encounter. For each type, you learn the best way to display and communicate results. You'll learn what analyses need to be performed, what tables and figures should be generated, and what statistical procedures should be employed for the analysis.

You'll walk step by step through the preparation of a typical final report. And you'll learn how to detect and avoid common errors in analysis and interpretation. A glossary of statistical terms is provided for help in decoding your statistician's reports.

REPORT COVERAGE

In this section we consider what material should be displayed and analyzed.

Each of the reports you prepare, from a brief abstract to the final comprehensive report, should cover the following topics:

- **Study population**
- **Baseline values**
- **Intermediate snapshots**
- **Protocol deviations**
- **Final results**
  — Primary end points
  — Adverse events
  — Other secondary end points

A Manager's Guide to the Design and Conduct of Clinical Trials, by Phillip I. Good
Copyright ©2006 John Wiley & Sons, Inc.

The final comprehensive report also will have to include

1. Demonstrations of similarities and differences for the following:
   - Baseline values of the various treatment groups
   - Data from the various treatment sites
   - End points of the various subgroups determined by baseline variables and adjunct therapies.
2. Explanations of protocol deviations including
   - Ineligible patients who were accidentally included in the study
   - Missing data
   - Dropouts and withdrawals
   - Modifications to treatment

Further explanations and stratifications will be necessary if the frequencies of any of the protocol deviations differ among treatments. For example, if there are differences in the baseline demographics of the treatment groups, then subsequent results will need to be stratified accordingly. If one or two sites stand out from the rest, then the results from these must be analyzed separately. Moreover, some plausible explanation for the differences must be advanced.

Here is another example. Suppose the vast majority of women in the study were in the control group. Then, to avoid drawing false conclusions about the men, the results for men and women must be presented separately unless one first can demonstrate that the treatments have similar effects on men and women.

UNDERSTANDING DATA

The way in which we present the data to be used in our reports and the methods of analysis we employ depend upon the type of data that is involved.

As noted in Chapter 6, data may be divided into three categories:

1. Categorical data such as sex and race
2. Metric observations such as age where differences and ratios are meaningful
3. Ordinal data such as subjective ratings of improvement, which may be viewed either as ordered categories or as discrete metric data depending on the context.

In this preliminary section, we consider how we would go about displaying and analyzing each of these data types.

Categories

When we only have two categories as is the case with sex, we would report the number in one of the categories, the total number of

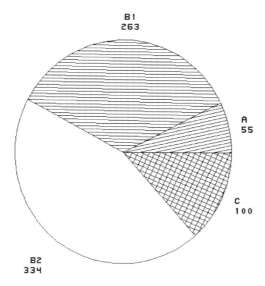

FIGURE 15.1 Pie chart depicts relative proportions of patients in the various ACA/AHA classifications. Actual frequencies are also displayed.

meaningful observations, and the percentage as in "170 of 850 patients or 20% were females."

When we have four or more categories the results are best summarized in the form of a pie chart as in Figure 15.1. Or, if we wish to make comparisons among multiple treatment groups, in the form of a banded bar chart as in Figure 15.2.

If there are only two treatments, we might also want to report a confidence interval for the *odds ratio* defined as $p_2(1 - p_1)/p_1(1 - p_2)$ where p_1 is the probability a subject in the first treatment group will belong to the first category and p_2 is a similar probability for the second treatment group.

If $p_2 = p_1$, the odds ratio is 1. If $p_2 > p_1$, the odds ratio is greater than 1. If the *confidence interval* for the odds ratio includes 1, e.g., (0.98, 1.02), we

> **CONFIDENCE INTERVALS**
>
> Bosses always want a bottom line number. But the probability is zero that any single value based on clinical data will be correct. When caught between a boss and a hard place, the solution is to provide an interval, e.g., (0.98, 1.02), you can guarantee with confidence will cover the correct value 90% or 95% of the time. As you might expect, the more precise and the greater the number of observations you make, the narrower that confidence interval will be.

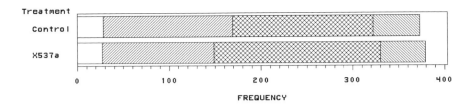

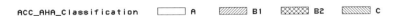

FIGURE 15.2 Bar chart depicts relative proportions of patients in the various ACA/AHA classifications. Actual frequencies are also displayed.

will have no reason to believe the two treatments have different effects on the variable we are studying.

Metric Data

For metric data such as age, we would normally report both the arithmetic mean of the sample and the standard error of the mean, for example 59.3 ± 0.55 years, along with the sample size, n = 350.

If the data take the form of a time to an event, it is more common to report the median or halfway point and to display the entire distribution in graphic form.

Report All Values with the Appropriate Degree of Precision.

Many computer programs yield values with eight or nine decimal places, most of which are meaningless. For example, because we can only measure age to the nearest day, it would be foolish to report mean age as 59.3724 years.

Even though we can measure age to the nearest day, it also would be foolish to report the mean age as 59.31 years, when the *standard error* is 0.55. The standard error is a measure of the *precision* of our estimate. It tells us how close we are likely to come to our original estimate if we repeat the sampling process many times.

If the underlying population has the form of a bell-shaped curve depicted in Figure 6.1, then in 95% of the samples we would expect the sample mean to lie within two standard errors of the mean of our original sample.

Increasing the sample size decreases the standard error, reflecting the increase in precision of the mean. By taking four times as many

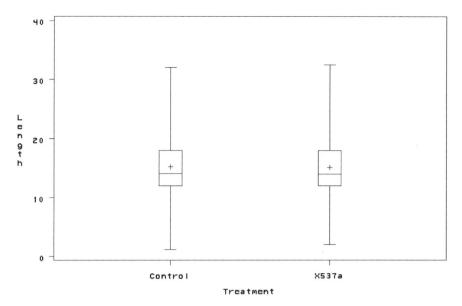

FIGURE 15.3 Box and Whiskers Plot. The box encompasses the middle 50% of each sample while the "whiskers" indicate the smallest and largest values. The line through the box is the median of the sample, that is, 50% of the sample is larger than this value, while 50% is smaller. The asterisk indicates the sample mean. Note that the mean is shifted in the direction of a small number of very large values.

observations, we can cut the standard error in half. Had we made tens of thousands of observations in our hypothetical example, we would have been able to report the mean value as 59.31 ± 0.055.

The standard error is not a measure of *accuracy*. I remember a cartoon depicting Robin Hood, bow in hand, examining where his arrows had each split the arrow in front of it. Unfortunately, all three arrows had hit a cow rather than the deer he was aiming at. The mean may not provide a valid representation of the center of the population when the observations do not come from a symmetric distribution such as that depicted in Figure 6.1.

When the data do not come from a symmetric distribution, it is preferable to report the median or 50th percentile along with the range and the 25th and 75th percentiles. Because it's hard to grasp such information in text form, a box and whiskers plot such as that in Figure 15.3 provides the most effective way to present the data and to make a comparison between the two treatment groups.

> **CHOOSING THE RIGHT STATISTIC**
>
> At first glance, it would seem that statistics as a branch of mathematics ought to be an exact science and the choice of the correct statistical procedure determined automatically. But at least four influences are at work:
>
> 1. **Accuracy.** The p-value or significance level determined by a statistical method is correct (that is exact or accurate) only if the assumptions underlying the method are satisfied.
> 2. **Computational Feasibility.** Rapid advances in hardware and software technology have made all but the most intractable of statistical methods practical today.
> 3. **Regulatory Agency Requirements.** The members of the various committees who exercise oversight on behalf of the regulatory agency must be satisfied with the statistical methods that are used. Although counterarguments often fall on deaf ears, committee "recommendations" can often be forestalled by providing appropriate justification for the statistical techniques that are utilized, particularly when such techniques are a relatively recent introduction in the analysis of clinical trials.
> 4. **Familiarity.** Too often, the choice of statistical method is determined on the basis of the technique that was used in the last set of clinical trials or the limited subset of techniques with which the biostatistician is familiar.
>
> The fact that a method was not rejected in the past is no guarantee that it will not be rejected in the future. Regulatory agencies are composed of individuals. What one individual or individuals once found acceptable may meet with rejection by their replacements.
>
> The only safety lies with carefully chosen, proven statistical methodology.

If there are only two treatments, we might also want to report a confidence interval for the difference in mean values. If this confidence interval includes zero, we would infer that the treatments have approximately the same effect on the variable we are studying.

Ordinal Data. When we have a small number of ordered categories (12 or less), the data should be reported in tabular form. Otherwise, report as you would metric data.

STATISTICAL ANALYSIS

How we conduct the analysis of the final results will depend upon whether or not

- **Baseline results of the treatment groups are equivalent.**
- **Results of the disparate treatment sites may be combined.**
- **Results of the various adjunct treatment groups may be combined. (if adjunct treatments were used).**
- **Proportions of missing data, dropouts and withdrawals are unrelated to treatment.**

TABLE 15.1 Sandoz Results by Test Site

Test Site	New Drug		Control Drug	
	Responded	N	Responded	N
2	0	39	6	32
3	1	20	3	18
4	1	14	2	15
5	1	20	2	19
6	0	12	2	10
7	3	49	10	2
8	0	19	2	17
9	1	14	0	15
10	2	26	2	27
11	0	19	2	18
12	0	12	1	11
13	0	24	5	19
14	2	10	2	11
15	0	14	11	3
16	0	53	4	48
19	1	50	1	48
20	0	13	1	13
21	0	13	1	13

Thus the first steps in our analysis must be to address these issues.

Consider the results summarized in Table 15.1 obtained by the Sandoz drug company and reproduced with permission from the StatXact manual. Obviously, the results of sites 20 and 21 are the same, but are they the same as at the other sites? And what of site 15 with its extraordinarily large number of responses in the control group. Can the results for site 15 be combined with the results for the other sites? As it turns out, an analysis of this data shows that there are statistically significant differences.

The analysis of a metric end point to determine whether the data from various subsets may be combined usually takes the form of a *t-test* or an *analysis of variance* as in the sample output in Figure 15.4.

If we can resolve all the above issues in the negative, then the analysis is straightforward. Otherwise, we need to subdivide the sample into strata based on the differentiating factors and perform a separate analysis for each stratum.

Stratification may sometimes be necessitated even when the differences occasioned by differences in treatment are not statistically significant. See the section headed "Simpson's Paradox" later on in this chapter.

A recent clinical study illustrates some of the complications that can arise. Significant differences were found in the proportions of

```
Dependent Variable: Restenosis
                                       Sum of
Source                  DF           Squares     Mean Square    F Value    Pr > F
Model                    7         1950.0286        278.5755       0.67    0.7002
Error                  530       221409.8899        417.7545
Corrected Total        537       223359.9185

                 R-Square       Coeff Var       Root MSE     Restenosis Mean
                 0.008730        55.00208       20.43904     37.16049

Source                  DF       Type III SS    Mean Square    F Value    Pr > F
adjunct                  1        117.086311     117.086311       0.28    0.5967
gndr                     1         17.599391      17.599391       0.04    0.8375
adjunct*gndr             1          3.513639       3.513639       0.01    0.9270
treat                    1        749.289470     749.289470       1.79    0.1811
adjunct*treat            1       1630.494191    1630.494191       3.90    0.0487
gndr*treat               1        258.062879     258.062879       0.62    0.4322
adjunct*gndr*treat       1        417.994484     417.994484       1.00    0.317
```

FIGURE 15.4 Results of a SAS Analysis of the Joint Effects of Gender, Adjunct Therapy, and Treatment on Restenosis. The significance level (Pr > F) is less than 0.5 for just one of the terms above,[40] suggesting that the effect of adjunctive therapy on restenosis varies between the two treatment groups. A further detailed breakdown of the results revealed that while the adjunct therapy had a positive effect in the control group, its use was contradicted in the presence of the experimental treatment.

men and women that had been assigned to the various treatment groups. Exacerbating the situation was the discovery that men and women reacted differently to the adjuvant treatment.

The final results were broken out separately by men and women and whether they'd received the adjuvant or not (Table 15.2). One hundred percent of the women in the control group who received the adjuvant recovered completely, a totally unexpected result!

The adjuvant treatment also was of positive value for the men in the control group, but appeared to inhibit healing and was of negative value for those men who received the experimental treatment.

Categorical Data

Comparisons of categorical data may be displayed in the form of a contingency table. (Tables 15.1 and 15.3) In a 2 × 2 table such as that of Table 15.3 the recommended analysis is Fisher's exact test. For a comparison of the odds ratios at various treatment sites as in Table 15.1, the recommended test is based on the permutation distribution of the Zelen statistic.

The chi-square distribution was used in the past to determine the significance level of both tables, although it was well known that the

---

[40]As we discuss further in what follows, these probabilities are at best approximations to the actual significance levels.

TABLE 15.2 Binary Stenosis by Adjunct, Gender, and Treatment

Adjunct	Gender	NuStent		Standard		p
		N	Mean	N	Mean	
No	M	143	24	149	27	0.68
	F	51	26	42	24	0.97
Yes	M	67	28	60	17	0.15
	F	15	47	19	0	0.001

TABLE 15.3 Subset Analysis

	Full Recovery	Impairment
With adjunct	11	0
Without adjunct	17	5

chi-square distribution was only a poor approximation to the actual distribution of these statistics. For example, an analysis of Table 15.3 yields a p-value of 4.3% based on the chi-square distribution and Pearson's chi-square statistic, whereas the correct and exact p-value as determined by Fisher's method is 11.1%. An analysis of Table 15.1 yields a p-value of 7.8% based on the chi-square distribution, yet the correct and exact p-value as determined from the permutation distribution of Zelen's statistic is a highly significant 1.2%.

Today, methods that yield exact and correct p-values for virtually every form of contingency table are available. See Mehta and Patel (1998), Mehta, Patel, and Tsiatis (1984), and Good (2005; Chapter 6). Yet many statisticians continue to utilize the erroneous chi-square approximation, much like a drunk might search for his missing wallet under the lamp post because the light there was better.

Ordinal Data

We often deal with data that are ordered but nonmetric, such as self-evaluation scales. The observations can be ordered because "much improved" is obviously superior to merely "improved," but they are nonmetric because we cannot add and subtract the observations. To see that this is true, ask yourself whether one patient who is "much improved" and a second patient who shows "no change" are equivalent to two patients who are merely "improved"?

Such data have often been analyzed by chi-square methods as well. But a chi-square analysis is really a multisided test designed to detect any and all alternatives to the null hypothesis rather than being

TABLE 15.4 Adverse Events per Patient by Treatment

	0	1	2	3	4	5	6	7	8	9	10	11	13
New	233	56	30	21	16	5	7	6	2	2	1	1	0
Standard	253	46	28	17	13	4	2	3	0	1	1	0	1

focused against the single ordered alternative of interest. The result is that the chi-square analysis is not very powerful. If we were to analyze the data of Table 15.4 using the chi-square statistic, we would obtain a *p*-value of 0.51 and conclude there was no significant difference between the two treatments. But if we note that the columns in the table are ordered from patients with no adverse events to patients with as many as 13 and use the Wilcoxon rank test, we obtain a highly significant *p*-value of 0.025.[41]

Metric Data

Statistics is an evolving science. Statisticians are always trying to develop new and more powerful statistical techniques that will make the most from the data at hand.

Virtually all statistical tests employed in clinical trials require that

1. Patients be drawn at random from the population
2. Patients be assigned at random to treatment
3. Observations on different patients be independent of one another
4. Under the hypothesis of no treatment differences, *the null hypothesis*, all the observations in the samples being compared come from the same distribution.[42]

Parametric methods also require that the observations come from a normal distribution, that is, a bell-shaped curve similar to the one depicted in Figure 6.1. Thus nonparametric tests, which do not have this restriction are usually to be preferred to parametric for the analysis of metric data.

Examples of *parametric* methods include the *t*-test for comparing means and the F-test used in the analysis of variance. The F-test provides exact *p*-values if all the above restrictions are met.

But even with only moderate deviations from the bell-shaped

---

[41] Even this Patter test may be improved upon; see Berger, Permutt, and Ivanova (1998).
[42] Implicit to this assumption is that the patients have been randomly assigned to treatment.

normal distribution, the *p*-values provided by the F-test can be quite misleading (see Good & Lunneborg, 2005). The *t*-test is more robust and provides almost exact *p*-values for most samples of metric data larger than ten in number.[43]

Examples of *nonparametric* methods include permutation tests based on ranks, such as the Wilcoxon test for comparing two samples and the Kruskall-Wallace test for comparing k-samples, and permutation tests based on the original observations. These tests always provide exact significance levels if the two basic assumptions of independence and equal variances are satisfied.

Permutation tests based on the original observations are more powerful and should be used in preference to rank tests unless there is reason to believe the data may contain one or more *outliers* (exceptional values or typographical errors). Ranks diminish the effects of outliers. For example, the mean of 1.1, 2.2, 3.4, 4.3, 59 is 14; taking ranks, the mean of 1, 2, 3, 4, 5 is 3.

Software providing for permutation tests based on the original observations has been in short supply until recently. Today, permutation software is available for comparing two samples, for comparing k-samples with either ordered or unordered categories, and for the analysis of multifactor designs.

A second weakness of the parametric analysis of variance approach is that it only provides for a test of the null or no-difference-in-effect hypothesis against all possible alternatives. If we know in advance that the alternative has a specific form (an ordered dose response, for example), then one can always find a more powerful permutation test to take advantage of this knowledge. For more on this topic, see Salsburg (1992).

An Example

Owning a statistics program no more make you a statistician than buying a pamphlet called "Brain Surgery Made Easy" will turn you into a neurosurgeon. Although almost anyone can learn to use a statistics program (or a scalpel), interpreting the results is quite a different matter. Consider the output of one of the less complex of SAS's many statistics routines, the *t*-test procedure.

---

[43] Of course, one easily can find extreme cases that are an exception to this rule.

```
                      The TTEST Procedure
                           Statistics

                        Lower          Upper
                        CL             CL          Lower CL              Upper CL
Variable treat   N      Mean   Mean    Mean    Std Dev Std Dev Std Dev   Std Err
RIG      New     121   0.5527 0.5993  0.6459   0.2299  0.2589  0.2964    0.0235
RIG      Stand   127   0.5721 0.598   0.6238   0.1312  0.1474  0.1681    0.0131
RIG      Diff (1-2)   -0.051  0.0013  0.0537   0.1924  0.2093  0.2296    0.0266

                            T-Tests

Variable    Method              Variances       DF      t Value      Pr > |t|
RIG         Pooled              Equal           246     0.05         0.9608
RIG         Satterthwaite       Unequal         188     0.05         0.9613

                       Equality of Variances

Variable    Method          Num DF      Den DF      F Value       Pr > F
RIG         Folded F        120         126         3.09          <.0001
```

The first table of the SAS output provides us with confidence limits for the mean and standard deviation of the variable RIG for each of the two treatment groups. We would report the results as RIG is 0.59 ± 0.02 for those receiving the new treatment and 0.59 ± 0.01 for those receiving the standard.

There does not appear to be a significant difference between the RIG values of the two treatments, for the *t*-value is quite small and the probability of observing a larger *t*-value by chance is 0.96 or close to 1. However, because the variances are significantly different (as shown in the last row of the output) the results of the *t*-test shown in the second table cannot be relied on.[44]

Time-To-Event Data

Possible events for which you might wish to track the time after treatment to include "symptom free," "recurrence of symptoms," and "death." Although survival or time-to-event data are metric (or at least ordinal), the presentation and analysis of results take on a quite different character. If the events are inevitable and the trials last long enough, then we can compare treatments as we do with metric data, using either a permutation test applied to the original observations or, if we want to diminish the effects of a few very lengthy time intervals, the ranks of the observations in the combined sample.[45]

---

[44]Details of the correct statistical procedure to use with unequal variances, known as the Behrens-Fisher problem, are given later in this chapter.

[45]Tests based on a normal distribution would not be appropriate as the distribution is far from normal, the mean "time-to-event" typically being much greater than the median.

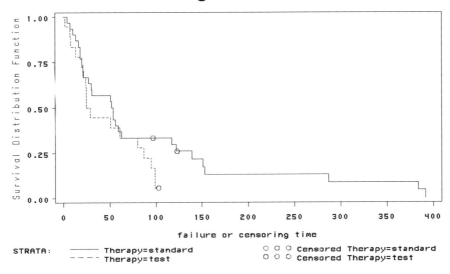

FIGURE 15.5 Depicting Time-to-Event Data with the Aid of a Survival Curve.

But time-to-event data are often censored; for many of the patients, the event being tracked may have not yet occurred by the time the trials end, so only a minimum value can be recorded. A graph such as Figure 15.5 is the most effective way to present the results. The circles denote those observations that are censored; they represent times that might have been much longer had the trials been allowed to continue.

In most animal experiments, all the subjects receive the treatment on the same date and are subject to the same degree of censoring. The optimal statistic, described by Good (1992), takes into account both the time-to-event for those animals in which the event occurred during the study period and the relative proportions between treatments of animals that complete the trials without the event occurring.

In trials with humans, patients are enrolled on an ongoing basis. One patient may be followed for several years, and another may be enrolled in the trials only a few months before they end. Patients who enter the study long after the trials have begun are more likely to have small recorded values. This is one of the reasons why we often specify two cut-off dates for trials, one denoting the last date on which a patient may enter the study and the more recent representing the date on which the last observation will be made.

TABLE 15.5 SAS Output from an Analysis Using Proc Lifetest

Univariate Chi-Squares for the Wilcoxon Test				
Variable	Test Statistic	Standard Deviation	Chi-Square	Pr > Chi-Square
Treatment	-1.9670	1.9399	1.0281	0.3106
Univariate Chi-Squares for the Log-Rank Test				
Variable	Test Statistic	Standard Deviation	Chi-Square	Pr > Chi-Square
Treatment	-4.3108	2.8799	2.2405	0.1344
Forward Stepwise Sequence of Chi-Squares for the Wilcoxon Test				
Variable	DF	Chi-Square	Pr > Chi-Square	Chi-Square Increment	Pr > Increment
Karnofsky index	1	11.0918	0.0009	11.0918	0.0009
Treatment	2	11.4047	0.0033	0.3128	0.5759
Forward Stepwise Sequence of Chi-Squares for the Log-Rank Test				
Variable	DF	Chi-Square	Pr > Chi-Square	Chi-Square Increment	Pr > Increment
Karnofsky index	1	5.4953	0.0191	5.4953	0.0191
Treatment	2	7.9177	0.0191	2.4224	0.1196

> **TYPES OF DATA**
>
> Binomial—The observations fall into one of two categories, heads vs. tails, success vs. failure, yes vs. no.
>
> Categorical—The data are subdivided into categories such as black, white, Hispanic.
>
> Ordinal—The observations can be ordered from smallest to largest (though there may be ties). Examples include rating scales.
>
> Metric—Ordinal data for which the differences between observations are meaningful. Examples include age, height, and percent stenosis.
>
> Survival—Data for which the time to the event is recorded. Examples include survival time, time to relapse, and time till the absence of a symptom or symptoms.

A different form of analysis is called for, one that imputes values to the censored observations based on a mathematical model. The two principal methods are a log-rank test and a test based on a censored Wilcoxon.

Generally, the log-rank test should be employed if the emphasis is to be placed on early time-to-event data. The results for the data depicted in Figure 15.5 are given in Table 15.5. The large p-value of 0.3 or 30% reveals that treatment does not have a significant effect on survival.

In many cases, one would also want to correct for cofactors. The second part of Table 15.5 reveals the statistically significant relation of survival to the Karnofsky Index, which is a measure of the overall status of the cancer patient at the time of entry into the clinical trials.

STEP BY STEP

The guidelines presented here are generic; always consult the current guidelines published by the cognizant regulatory agency before beginning or submitting the results of a statistical analysis. A copy of the 1996 IHS Guideline for the Format and Content of the Clinical and Statistical Sections of an Application may be downloaded from *http://www.fda.gov/cder/guidance/statnda.pdf*.

The purpose of the statistical analysis section of the final report like that of the final report itself is tell a story in as clear and concise a fashion as possible. Only the tabular material and graphs associated with the main theme should be incorporated directly in the analysis section. All the other material described in what follows should be deferred to appendixes.

The Study Population

Begin by describing the study population in terms of the eligibility criteria, the proportion of males and females, average age of the participants and so forth. For categorical variables such as sex and race, report both the percentages and numbers in each category. For continuous variables such as age, report the mean, standard error of the mean and sample size.

Note that sample and subsample sizes are always based on the number of patients, not on the number of eyes or tumors or teeth or injuries that may have been treated. This is true even if the individual organs have been treated independently of one another.

A side-by-side comparison of baseline values should be provided in tabular form as in Table 15.6. Include confidence limits, but do not include *p*-values. In the opinion of Lang and Secic (1997), "Clinical imbalances, even though the result of chance, are real and need to be accounted for in the subsequent analysis. Statistical comparisons of baseline values are rarely necessary.

"Statistically significant differences will be the result of chance [because of the large number of simultaneous tests that are being performed], and nonstatistically significant differences do not indicate

TABLE 15.6 Baseline Comparison

	New, $N = 380$	Standard, $N = 370$	Odds Ratio
Men	74%	78%	0.80 (0.57, 1.12)
Diabetes	36%	35%	0.96 (0.70, 1.30)
Current Smoker	28%	29%	1.04 (0.75, 1.44)
Elev Cholesterol	58%	58%	0.99 (0.73, 1.34)
Hypertension	59%	54%	0.80 (0.60, 1.09)

that the groups are comparable, but rather that randomization was effective."

See also Altman and Dore (1990).

Show that the results of the various treatment sites can be combined. If the endpoint is binary in nature—success vs. failure—employ Zelen's (1971) test of equivalent odds ratios in 2×2 tables. If it appears that one or more treatment sites should be excluded, provide a detailed explanation for the exclusion if possible ("repeated protocol violations," "ineligible patients," "no control patients," "misdiagnosis") and exclude these sites from the subsequent analysis.[46]

Determine which baseline and environmental factors, if any, are correlated with the primary end point. Perform a statistical test to see whether there is a differential effect between treatments as a result of these factors.

Test to see whether there is a differential effect on the end point between treatments occasioned by the use of any adjunct treatments.

Reporting Primary End Points

Report the results for each primary end point separately. For each end point:

1. **Report the aggregate results by treatment for all patients who were examined during the study.**
2. **Report the aggregate results by treatment only for those patients who were actually eligible, who were treated originally as randomized, or who were not excluded for any other reason. Provide significance levels for treatment comparisons.**
3. **Break down these latter results into subsets based on factors predetermined before the start of the study such as adjunct therapy or gender. Provide significance levels for treatment comparisons.**
4. **List all factors uncovered during the trials that appear to have altered the effects of treatment. Provide a tabular comparison by treatment for these factors, but do not include *p*-values.**

If there were multiple end points, you have the option of providing a further multivariate comparison of the treatments.

Exceptions

Every set of large-scale clinical trials has its exceptions. You must report the raw numbers of such exceptions and, in some instances,

---

[46]Any explanation is bound to trigger inquiries from the regulatory agency. This is yet another reason why continuous monitoring of results and subsequent early remedial action is essential.

provide additional analyses that analyze or compensate for them. Typical exceptions include the following:

Did Not Participate. Subjects who were eligible and available but did not participate in the study—This group should be broken down further into those who were approached but chose not to participate and those who were not approached.

Ineligibles. In some instances, depending on the condition being treated, it may have been necessary to begin treatment before ascertaining whether the subject was eligible to participate in the study.

For example, an individual arrives at a study center in critical condition; the study protocol calls for a series of tests, the results of which may not be back for several days, but in the opinion of the examining physician treatment must begin immediately. The patient is randomized to treatment, and only later is it determined that the patient is ineligible.

The solution is to present two forms of the final analysis, one incorporating all patients, the other limited to those who were actually eligible.

Withdrawals. Subjects who enrolled in the study but did not complete it. Includes both dropouts and noncompliant patients. These patients might be subdivided further based on the point in the study at which they dropped out.

At issue is whether such withdrawals were treatment related. For example, the gastrointestinal side effects associated with erythromycin are such that many patients (including me) may refuse to continue with the drug.

If possible, subsets of both groups should be given detailed followup examinations to determine whether the reason for the withdrawal was treatment related.

Crossovers. If the design provided for intent to treat, a noncompliant patient may still continue in the study after being reassigned to an alternate treatment. Two sets of results should be reported: one for all patients who completed the trials (retaining their original assignments) and one only for those patients who persisted in the groups to which they were originally assigned.

Missing Data. Missing data are common, expensive, and preventable in many instances.

The primary end point of a recent clinical study of various cardiovascular techniques was based on the analysis of follow-up angiograms. Although more than 750 patients had been enrolled in the study, only 523 had the necessary angiograms. Put another way, almost a third of the monies spent on the trials had been wasted.

Missing data are often the result of missed follow-up appointments. The recovering patient no longer feels the need to return or, at the other extreme, is too sick to come into the physician's office. Non-compliant patients are also likely to skip visits.

You need to analyze the data to ensure that the proportions of missing observations are the same in all treatment groups. If the observations are critical, involving primary or secondary end points as in the preceding example, then you will need to organize a follow-up survey of at least some of the patients with missing data. Such surveys are extremely expensive.

As always, prevention is the best and sometimes the only way to limit the impact of missing data.

- **Ongoing monitoring and tying payment to delivery of critical documents are essential.**
- **Site coordinators on your payroll rather than the investigator's are more likely to do immediate follow-up when a patient does not appear at the scheduled time.**
- **A partial recoupment of the missing data can be made by conducting a secondary analysis based on the most recent follow-up value. See, Pledger [1992].**

A chart such as that depicted in Figure 15.6 is often the most effective way to communicate all this information; see, for example, Lang and Secic, [1997; p22].

Outliers. Suspect data such as that depicted in Figure 14.2. You may want to perform two analyses, one incorporating all the data, and one deleting the suspect data. A further issue is whether the proportion of suspect data is the same for all treatment groups.

Competing Events. A death or a disabling accident, whether or not it is directly related to the condition being treated, may prevent us from obtaining the information we need. The problem is a common one in long-term trials in the elderly or high-risk populations and is best compensated for by taking a larger than normal sample.

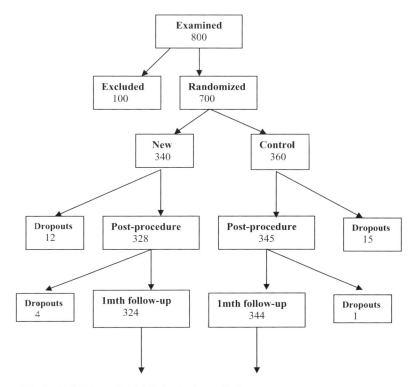

FIGURE 15.6 Where Did All the Patients Go?

Adverse Events

Report the number, percentage, and type of adverse events associated with each treatment. Accompany this tabulation with a statistical analysis of the set of adverse events as a whole as well as supplementary analyses of classes of adverse events that are known from past studies to be treatment or disease specific. If p-values are used, they should be corrected for the number of tests; see Westall and Young (1993) and Westall, Krishnen, and Young (1998).

Report the incidence of adverse events over time as a function of treatment. Detail both changes in the total number of adverse events and in the number of patients who remain incident free. You may also wish to distinguish various levels of severity.

ANALYTICAL ALTERNATIVES

In this section, we consider some of the more technically challenging statistical issues on which statisticians often cannot agree including a) unequal variances, b) testing for equivalence, c) Simpson's paradox, and d) estimating precision.

When Statisticians Can't Agree

Statistics is not an exact science. Nothing demonstrates this more than the Behrens-Fisher problem of unequal variances in the treatment groups. Recall that the t-test for comparing results in two treatment groups is valid only if the variances in the two groups are equal. Statisticians do not agree on which statistical procedure should be used if they are not. When I submitted this issue recently to a group of experienced statisticians, almost everyone had their own preferred method. Here is just a sampling of the choices:

- t-test. One statistician commented, "SAS PROC TTEST is nice enough to present p-values for both equal and unequal variances. My experience is that the FDA will always accept results of the t-test without the equal variances assumption—they would rather do this than think."
- Wilcoxon test. The use of the ranks in the combined sample reduces the impact (though it does not eliminate the effect) of the difference in variability between the two samples.
- Generalized Wilcoxon test. See O'Brien (1988).
- Procedure described in Manly and Francis (1999).
- Procedure described in Chapter 7 of Weerahandi (1995).
- Procedure described in Chapter 10 of Pesarin (2001).
- Bootstrap. Draw the bootstrap samples independently from each sample; compute the mean and variance of each bootstrap sample. Derive a confidence interval for the t-statistic.

Hilton (1996) compared the power of the Wilcoxon test, O'Brien test, and the Smirnov test in the presence of both location shift and scale (variance) alternatives. As the relative influence of the difference in variances grows, the O'Brien test is most powerful. The Wilcoxon test loses power in the face of different variances. If the variance ratio is 4:1, the Wilcoxon test is virtually useless.

One point is unequivocal. William Anderson writes, "The first issue is to understand *why* the variances are so different, and what does this mean to the patient. It may well be the case that a new treatment is not appropriate because of higher variance, even if the difference in means is favorable. This issue is important whether or not the difference was anticipated. Even if the regulatory agency does not raise the issue, I want to do so internally."

David Salsburg agrees. "If patients have been assigned at random to the various treatment groups, the existence of a significant different in any parameter of the distribution suggests that there is a difference in treatment effect. The problem is not how to compare the means but how to determine what aspect of this difference is relevant to the purpose of the study.

"Since the variances are significantly different, I can think of two situations where this might occur:

1. **In many clinical measurements there are minimum and maximum values that are possible, e.g., the Hamilton Depression Scale, or the number of painful joints in arthritis. If one of the treatments is very effective, it will tend to push patient values into one of the extremes. This will produce a change in distribution from a relatively symmetric one to a skewed one, with a corresponding change in variance.**
2. **The patients may represent a mixture of populations. The difference in variance may occur because the effective treatment is effective for only a subset of the patient population. A locally most powerful test is given in Conover and Salsburg (1988)."**

Testing for Equivalence

The statistical procedures for testing for statistical significance and for equivalence are quite different in nature.

The difference between the observations arising from two treatments T and C is judged *statistically significant* if it can be said with confidence level α that the difference between the mean effects of the two treatments is greater than zero.

Another way of demonstrating precisely the same thing is to show $c_L \leq 0 \leq c_R$ where c_L and c_R are the left and right boundaries respectively of a $1-2\alpha$ confidence interval for the difference in treatment means.

The value of α is taken most often to be 5%. ($\alpha = 10\%$ is sometimes used in preliminary studies.) In some instances, such as ruling out adverse effects, 1% or 2% may be required.

Failure to conclude significance does not mean that the variables are equal, or even equivalent. It may merely be the result of a small sample size. If the sample size is large enough, any two variables will be judged significantly different.

The difference between the variables arising from two treatments T and C will be judged will be called *equivalent* if the difference between the mean effects of the two treatments is less than a value Δ, called the *minimum relevant difference*.

This value Δ is chosen based on clinical, engineering, or scientific reasoning. There is no traditional mathematical value.

TABLE 15.7 Equivalence vs. Statistical Significance

	−	Δ	0	+	Δ
Equivalent Not Statistically Significant			(		)
Equivalent Statistically Significant				(	)
Not Equivalent Not Statistically Significant			(			)
Not Equivalent Statistically Significant				(		)

To perform a test of equivalence, we need to generate a confidence interval for the difference of the means:

1. Choose a sample from each group.
2. Construct a confidence interval for the difference of the means. For significance level α, this will be a 1–2α confidence interval.
3. If $-\Delta \leq c_L$ and $c_R \leq \Delta$, the groups are judged equivalent.

Table 15.7 depicts the left "(" and right ")" boundaries of such a confidence interval in a variety of situations.

Failure to detect a significance difference does not mean that the treatment effects are equal, or even equivalent. It may merely be the result of a small sample size. If the sample size is large enough, any two samples will be judged significantly different.

Simpson's Paradox

A significant p-value in the analysis of contingency tables only means that the variables are associated. It does not mean there is a cause and effect relationship between them. They may both depend on a third variable omitted from the study.

Regrettably, a third omitted variable may also result in two variables appearing to be independent when the opposite is true. Consider the following table, an example of what is termed Simpson's paradox:

	Population	
	Control	*Treated*
Alive	6	20
Dead	6	20

We don't need a computer program to tell us the treatment has no effect on the death rate. Or does it? Consider the following two tables that result when we examine the males and females separately:

	Males			Females	
	Control	Treated		Control	Treated
Alive	4	8	Alive	2	12
Dead	3	5	Dead	3	15

In the first of these tables, treatment reduces the male death rate from 0.43 to 0.38. In the second from 0.6 to 0.55. Both sexes show a reduction, yet the combined population does not. Resolution of this paradox is accomplished by avoiding a knee jerk response to statistical significance when association is involved. One needs to think deeply about underlying cause and effect relationships before analyzing data. Thinking about cause and effect relationships in the preceding example might have led us to thinking about possible sexual differences, and to testing for a common odds ratio.

Estimating Precision

Reporting results in terms of a mean and standard error as in 56 ± 3.2 is a long-standing tradition. Indeed, many members of regulatory committees would protest were you to do otherwise. Still, mathematical rigor and not tradition ought prevail when statistics is applied. Rigorous methods for estimating the precision of a statistic include the bias-corrected and accelerated bootstrap and the boostrap-t (Good, 2005a).

When metric observations come from a bell-shaped symmetric distribution, the probability is 95% on the average that the mean of the population lies within two standard errors of the sample mean. But if the distribution is not symmetric, as is the case when measurement errors are a percentage of the measurement, then a nonsymmetric interval is called for. One first takes the logarithms of the observations, computes the mean and standard error of the logarithms and determines a symmetric confidence interval. One then takes the antilogarithms of the boundaries of the confidence interval and uses these to obtain a confidence interval for the means of the original observations.

The drawback of the preceding method is that it relies on the assumption that the distribution of the logarithms is a bell-shaped distribution. If it is not, we're back to square one.

With the large samples that characterize long-term trials, the use of the *bootstrap* is always preferable. When we bootstrap, we treat the original sample as a stand-in for the population and resample from it repeatedly, 1000 times or so, with replacement, computing the average each time.

For example, here are the heights of a group of adolescents, measured in centimeters and ordered from shortest to tallest.

137.0 138.5 140.0 141.0 142.0 143.5 145.0 147.0 148.5 150.0 153.0 154.0 155.0 156.5 157.0 158.0 158.5 159.0 160.5 161.0 162.0 167.5

The median height lies somewhere between 153 and 154 centimeters. If we want to extend this result to the population, we need an estimate of the precision of this average.

Our first bootstrap sample, which I've arranged in increasing order of magnitude for ease in reading, might look like this:

138.5 138.5 140.0 141.0 141.0 143.5 145.0 147.0 148.5 150.0 153.0 154.0 155.0 156.5 157.0 158.5 159.0 159.0 159.0 160.5 161.0 162.

Several of the values have been repeated as we are sampling *with replacement*. The minimum of this sample is 138.5, higher than that of the original sample, the maximum at 162.0 is less than the original, while the median remains unchanged at 153.5.

137.0 138.5 138.5 141.0 141.0 142.0 143.5 145.0 145.0 147.0 148.5 148.5 150.0 150.0 153.0 155.0 158.0 158.5 160.5 160.5 161.0 167.5

In this second bootstrap sample, we again find repeated values; this time the minimum, maximum and median are 137.0, 167.5 and 148.5, respectively.

The medians of fifty bootstrapped samples drawn from our sample ranged between 142.25 and 158.25 with a median of 152.75 (see Fig. 15.7). They provide a feel for what might have been had we sampled repeatedly from the original population.

The bootstrap may also be used for tests of hypotheses. See, for example, Freedman et al. (1989) and Good (2005a, Chapter 2).

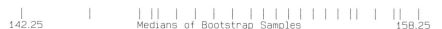

FIGURE 15.7 Scatterplot of 50 Bootstrap Medians Derived from a Sample of Heights.

BAD STATISTICS
Among the erroneous statistical procedures we consider in what follows are

- Using the wrong method
- Choosing the most favorable statistic
- Making repeated tests on the same data (which we also considered in chapter)
- Testing ad hoc, post hoc hypotheses

Using the Wrong Method
The use of the wrong statistical method—a large-sample approximation instead of an exact procedure, a multipurpose test instead of a more powerful one focused against specific alternatives, ordinary least-squares regression rather than Deming regression, or a test whose underlying assumptions are clearly violated—can, in most instances be attributed to what Peddiwell and Benjamin (1959) term the saber-tooth curriculum. Most statisticians were taught already outmoded statistical procedures and too many haven't caught up since.

A major recommendation for your statisticians (besides making sure they have copies of all my other books and regularly sign up for online courses at http://statistics.com) is that they remain current with evolving statistical practice. Continuing education, attendance at meetings and conferences directed at statisticians, as well as seminars at local universities and think tanks are musts. If the only texts your statistician has at her desk are those she acquired in graduate school, you're in trouble.

Deming Regression
Ordinary regression is useful for revealing trends or potential relationships. But in the clinical laboratory where both dependent and independent variables may be subject to variation, ordinary least-

---

STATISTIC CHECK LIST

Is the method appropriate to the type of data being analyzed?

Should the data be rescaled, truncated, or transformed prior to the analysis?

Are the assumptions for the test satisfied?

- Samples randomly selected
- Observations independent of one another
- Under the no-difference or null hypothesis, all observations come from the same theoretical distribution.
- (parametric tests) The observations come from a specific distribution.

Is a more powerful test statistic available?

squares regression methods are no longer applicable. A comparison of two methods of measurement is sure to be in error unless Deming (aka: errors-in-measurement) regression is employed. The leading article on this topic is Linnet (1998).

Choosing the Most Favorable Statistic

Earlier, we saw that one might have a choice of several different statistics in any given testing situation. Your choice should be spelled out in the protocol. It is tempting to choose among statistics and data transformations after the fact, selecting the one that yields or comes closest to yielding the desired result. Such a "choose-the-best" procedure will alter the stated significance level and is unethical.

Other illicit and unethical variations on this same theme include changing the significance level after the fact to ensure significant results (Moye, 2000, p. 149), using a one-tailed test when a two-tailed test is appropriate and vice versa (Moye, 2000, p. 145–148), and reporting p-values for after-the-fact subgroups (Good, 2003, p. 7–9, 13).

Making Repeated Tests on the Same Data

In the International Study of Infarct Survival (1988), patients born under the Gemini or Libra astrological birth signs did somewhat worse on aspirin than no aspirin in contrast to the apparent beneficial effects of aspirin on all other study participants.

Alas for those nutters of astrological bent, there is no hidden meaning in this result.

When we describe a test as significant at the 5% or 1 in 20 level, we mean that one in 20 times, we'll get a significant result by chance alone. That is, when we test to see whether there are any differences in the baseline values of the control and treatment groups, if we've made 20 different measurements, we can expect to see at least one statistically significant difference. This difference will not represent a flaw in our design but simply chance at work. To avoid this undesirable result—that is, to avoid making a type I error and attributing to a random event an effect where none exists, we have three alternatives:

1. **Using a stricter criteria for statistical significance, 1 in 50 times (2%) or 1 in 100 (1%) instead of 1 in 20 (5%)**
2. **Applying a correction factor such as that of Bonferroni that automatically applies a stricter significance level based on the number of tests we've made**

3. **Distinguishing between the hypotheses we began the study with (and accepting or rejecting these at the original significance level) while demanding additional corroborating evidence for those exceptional results (such as a dependence on astrological sign) that are uncovered for the first time during the trials**

Which alternative you adopt will depend upon the underlying situation.

If you have measured 20 or so study variables, then you will make 20 not-entirely-independent comparisons, and the Bonferroni inequality or the Westfall sequential permutation procedure is recommended.

If you are performing secondary analyses of relations observed after the data were collected, that is, relations not envisioned in the original design, then you have a right to be skeptical and to insist on either a higher significance level or to view the results as tentative requiring further corroboration.

A second example in which we have to modify rejection criteria is the case of adaptive testing that we considered in Chapter 14. To see why we cannot use the same values to determine statistical significance when we make multiple tests that we use for a single nonsequential test, consider a strategy many of adopt when we play with our children. It doesn't matter what the underlying game is—it could be a card game indoors with a small child, or a game of hoops out on the driveway with a teenager, the strategy is the same.

You are playing the best out of three games. If your child wins, you call it a day. If you win, you say let's play three out of five. If you win the next series, then you make it four out of seven and so forth. In most cases, by the time you quit, your child is able to say to his mother, "I beat daddy."[47]

Increasing the number of opportunities one has to win or to reject a hypothesis shifts the odds, so that to make the game fair again, or the significant level accurate, one has to shift the rejection criteria.

Ad Hoc, Post Hoc Hypotheses

Patterns in data can suggest but cannot confirm hypotheses unless these hypotheses were formulated before the data was collected.

Everywhere we look, there are patterns. In fact, the harder we look the more patterns we see. It is natural for us to want to attribute some underlying cause to these patterns. But those who have studied the laws of probability tell us that more often then not patterns are simply the result of random events.

---

[47]With teenagers, we sometimes try to make this strategy work in our favor.

Put another way, a cluster of events in time or in space has a greater probability than equally-spaced events. See, for example, Good (2005b, Section 3.3).

How can we determine whether an observed association represents an underlying cause and effect relationship or is merely the result of chance? The answer lies in the very controlled clinical trials we are conducting. When we set out to test a specific hypothesis, then the probability of a specific event is predetermined. But when we uncover an apparent association, one that may well have arisen purely by chance, we cannot be sure of the association's validity until we conduct a second set of controlled clinical trials.

Here are three examples taken (with suitable modifications to conceal their identity) from actual clinical trials.

1. Random, Representative Samples. The purpose of a recent set of clinical trials was to see whether a simple surgical procedure performed before taking a standard prescription medicine would improve blood flow and distribution in the lower leg.

The results were disappointing on the whole, but one of the marketing representatives noted that when a marked increase in blood flow was observed just after surgery, the long term prognosis was excellent. She suggested we calculate a p-value for a comparison of patients with an improved blood flow versus patients who had taken the prescription medicine alone.

Such a p-value would be meaningless. Only one of the two samples of patients in question had been taken at random from the population. The other sample was determined after the fact. An underlying assumption for all statistical tests is that in order to extrapolate the results from the sample in hand to a larger population, the samples must be taken at random from and be representative of that population.[48]

An examination of surgical procedures and of those characteristics which might forecast successful surgery definitely was called for. But the generation of a p-value and the drawing of any final conclusions has to wait on clinical trials specifically designed for that purpose.

2. Finding Predictors. A logistic regression reveals the apparent importance of certain unexpected factors in a trial's outcome including gender. A further examination of the data reveals that the 16 female patients treated with the standard therapy and the adjunct all

---

[48]See section 2.7 of Good (2005b) for a more detailed discussion.

realized a 100% recovery. Because of the small numbers of patients involved, and the fact that the effects of gender were not one of the original hypotheses, we cannot report a *p*-value. But we should consider launching a further set of trials targeted specifically at female patients.

We need to report all results to the regulatory agency separately by sex as well as with both sexes combined. We need to research the literature to see if there are prior reports of dependence on sex.[49] Not least, we need to perform a cost-benefit analysis to see if a set of clinical trials using a larger number of female subjects would be warranted. (See also Chapter 16.)

3. Adverse Events. We'd been fortunate in that only a single patient had died during the first six months of trials, when we received a report of a second death. Although, over 30 sites were participating in the trials, the second death was at the same clinic as the first! The deaths warranted an intensive investigation of procedures at that clinic even though we could not exclude the possibility that chance alone was at work.

INTERPRETATION

The last example in the preceding section illustrates the gap between statistical and clinical significance.

Statistical significance (also known as the *p*-value) is defined as the probability that an event might have occurred by chance alone. The smaller the probability, the more statistically significant the result is said to be.

Clinical significance is that aspect of a study's outcome that convinces physicians to modify or maintain their current practice of medicine.

Statistical significance can be a factor in determining clinical significance, but only if it occurs in conjunction with other clear and convincing evidence.[50]

Don't pad your reports and oral presentations with clinically insignificant findings. Do report statistically insignificant differences if this finding is of clinical significance.

Consider expressing the results of the primary outcome measures in the most clinically significant fashion. For example, on a practical

---

[49]We found that the original clinical trials of the adjunct had used only men.
[50]See http://www.indiana.edu/~stigtsts and MacKay and Oldford (2001) for more on this topic.

day-to-day level, it is the individual who concerns us, not the population. I don't care about mean blood levels when I have a headache, I want to know whether *my* headache will get better. The percentage of patients who experienced relief or a total cure will be more meaningful to me than any average.

For example, in reports on cardiovascular surgery, it is customary to report the rate of binary restenosis (occlusion of a coronary artery in excess of 50%) in the sample, along with the mean value for arterial occlusion.

DOCUMENTATION

As noted in previous chapters, the programs that can be used for interim analyses can also be used for analysis of the final results. Thus development of the programs used for analysis should begin at the same time as or just prior to completion of the programs used for data entry.

Two sets of programs are needed, one for the extraction of data and one for statistical analysis.

Insist on documentation of all computer programs used for data selection and analysis. Programmers as much or more as other staff in your employ tend to be highly mobile. You cannot rely on programmers who were with you during the early stages of the trials to be present at the trials' conclusion. Your staff should be encouraged to document during program development and to verify and enlarge on the documentation as each program is finalized.

A header similar to that depicted in Figure 15.8 should be placed at the start of each program. If the program is modified, the date and name of the person making the modification should be noted.

Project:	Crawfish
Program Name:	gender.sas
Programmer:	Donald Wood (March 2001/mod April/mod 7 Aug, 15 Aug)
Purpose:	Classifies patients by gender Lists patients for whom gender is unknown
Input:	pat_demg gndr_cd enroll2
Output:	genroll

FIGURE 15.8 The header briefly summarizes the essential information about each program including the name of the programmer, the program's purpose, the files it requires for input, and the files it creates.

TABLE 15.8 SAS Programs Used in the Analysis of Crawfish (does not include adhoc queries)

File Name	Developed by Donald Wood 13-Aug-01		
	Purpose	Input	Output
adverse	Calculates frequency of adverse events	adv_evnt random	mace
age02	Calculates age of patients; prints list of patno's with misg data.	pat_demg, smlsrg, enroll2	
angio	Computes average preprocedure lesion length Prints list of patients without CORE reports	angiolab random aetrtmt	

```
***Begin check for patients with missing gender
   data ***;
***This section makes a comparison of the two
   adjunct treatment groups ***;
```

Comments similar to these should precede each step in the program and the time required for documentation (about 10% of the time required for the program itself) should be incorporated in time lines and work assignments.

A summary table listing all programs should be maintained as in Table 15.8.

FOR FURTHER INFORMATION

Abramson NS; Kelsey SF; Dafra P; Sutton-Tyrell KS. (1992) Simpson's paradox and clinical trials: what you find is not necessarily what you prove. *Ann Emerg Med* 21:1480–1482.

Altman DG; Dore CJ. (1990) Randomisation and baseline comparisons in clinical trials. *Lancet* 335:149–153.

Bailar JC; Moseteller F. (1992) *Medical Uses of Statistics*. 2nd ed. Boston: NEJM Books.

Begg CB. (1990) Suspended judgment. Significance tests of covariance imbalance in clinical trials. *Control Clin Trials* 11:223–225.

Berger V; Permutt T; Ivanova A. (1998) The convex hull test or ordered categorical data. *Biometrics* 54:1541-1550.

Cleveland WS. (1984) Graphs in scientific publications. *Amer Statist* 38:261–269.

Conover W; Salsburg D. (1988) *Biometrics* 44:189–196.

Dar R; Serlin; Omer H. (1994) Misuse of statistical tests in three decades of psychotherapy research. *J. Consult Clin Psychol* 62:75–82.

Dmitrienko A, Molenberghs G, Chuang-Stein C, Offen W. (2005) *Analysis of Clinical Trials Using SAS: A Practical Guide*. SAS Publishing.

Donegani M. (1991) An adaptive and powerful test. *Biometrika* 78:930–933.

Entsuah AR. (1990) Randomization procedures for analyzing clinical trend data with treatment related withdrawals. *Comm Statist* A 19:3859–3880.

Feinstein AR. (1976) Clinical Biostatistics XXXVII. Demeaned errors, confidence games, nonplussed minuses, inefficient coefficients, and other statistical disruptions of scientific communication. *Clin Pharmacol Ther* 20:617–631.

Fienberg SE. (1990) Damned lies and statistics: misrepresentations of honest data. In: Editorial Policy Committee. *Ethics and Policy in Scientific Publications*. Council of Biology Editors. pp 202–206.

Freedman L; Sylvester R; Byar DP. (1989) Using permutation tests and bootstrap confidence limits to analyze repeated events data from clinical trials. *Control Clin Trials* 10:129–141.

Gail MH; Tan WY; Piantadosi S. (1988) Tests for no treatment effect in randomized clinical trials. *Biometrika* 75:57–64.

Good PI. (1992) Globally almost most powerful tests for censored data. *J Nonpar Statist* 1:253-262.

Good P. (2003) *Common Errors in Statistics and How to Avoid Them*. Wiley: NY.

Good P. (2005a) *Resampling Methods*, 3rd ed. Birkhauser: Boston.

Good PI. (2005b) *Introduction to Statistics via Resampling Methods and Microsoft Office Excel*®. Wiley: Hoboken.

Good PI; Lunneborg C. (2005) Limitations of the analysis of variance. *J Modern Appl Statist Methods* 4:(2).

Hilton J. (1996) *Statist Med* 15:631–645.

Howard M (pseud for Good P). (1981) Randomization in the analysis of experiments and clinical trials. *Am Lab* 13:98–102.

International Study of Infarct Survival Collaborative Group. (1988) Randomized trial of intravenous streptokinase, oral aspirin, both or neither, among 17187 cases of suspected acute myocardial infarction. ISIS-2. *Lancet* ii:349–362.

Lachin JM. (1988) Properties of sample randomization in clinical trials. *Contr Clin Trials* 9:312–326.

Lachin JM. (1988) Statistical properties of randomization in clinical trials. *Contr Clin Trials* 9:289–311.

Linnet K. (1998) Perfomance of Dming regression nalysis in cas of misspecified analytical error ration in method comparison studies. *Clin Chem* 44:1024–031.

MacKay RJ; Oldford RW. (2001) Scientific method, statistical method and the speed of light. *Statist Sci* 15:254–278.

Manly B; Francis C. (1999) Analysis of variance by randomization when variances are unequal. *Aust New Zeal J Statist* 41:411–430.

Mehta CR; Patel NR. (1998) Exact inference for categorical data. In *Encyclopedia of Statistics*. Wiley: Hoboken.

Mehta CR; Patel NR; Gray R. (1985) On computing an exact confidence interval for the common odds ratio in several 2 × 2 contingency tables. *JASA* 80:969–973.

Mehta CR; Patel NR; Tsiatis AA. (1984) Exact significance testing to establish treatment equivalence with ordered categorical data. *Biometrics* 40:819–825.

O'Brien P. (1988) Comparing two samples: extension of the t, rank-sum, and log-rank tests. *JASA* 83:52–61.

Oosterhoff J. (1969) *Combination of One-Sided Statistical Tests*. Mathematisch Centrum Amsterdam.

Peddiwell JA; Benjamin HH (1959) *Saber-Tooth Curriculum*. New York: McGraw-Hill Professional Publishing.

Pesarin F. (2001) *Multivariate Permutation Tests*. New York: Wiley.

Pledger GW. (1992) Basic statistics: importance of adherence. *J Clin Res Pharmacoepidemiol* 6:77–81.

Pothoff RF; Peterson BL; George SL. (2001) Detecting treatment-by-center interaction in multi-center clinical trials. *Statist Med* 20:193–213.

Salsburg DS. (1992) *The Use of Restricted Significance Tests in Clinical Trials*. New York: Springer-Verlag.

Shih JH; Fay MP. (1999) A class of permutation tests for stratified survival distributions. *Biometrics* 55:1156–1161.

Troendle JF; Blair RC; Rumsey D; Moke P. (1997) Parametric and non-parametric tests for the overall comparison of several treatments to a control when treatment is expected to increase variability. *Statist Med* 16:2729–2739.

Wears RI. (1994) What is necessary for proof? Is 95% sure unrealistic? [Letter] *JAMA* 271:272.

Weerahandi S. (1995) *Exact Statistical Methods for Data Analysis*. (Springer Verlag, Berlin).

Wei LJ; Smythe RT; Smith RL. (1986) K-treatment comparisons in clinical trials. *Annals Math Statist* 14:265–274.

Westall PH; Krishnen A; Young S. (1998) Using prior information to allocate significance levels for multiple endpoints. *Statist Med* 17:2107–2119.

Westfall PH; Young SS. (1993) *Resampling-Based Multiple Testing: Examples and Methods for p-value Adjustment*. New York: John Wiley.

Zelen M. (1971) The analysis of several 2 × 2 contingency tables. *Biometrika* 58:129–137.

A PRACTICAL GUIDE TO STATISTICAL TERMINOLOGY

Statisticians tend to utilize their own strange and often incomprehensible language. Here is a practical guide to the more commonly used terms. Italicized terms are included in this glossary.

Analysis of variance	A technique for analyzing data in which the effects of several factors are taken into account simultaneously such as treatment, sex, and the use of an adjunct treatment. *p-Values* obtained from this technique are often suspect as they rely on seldom realized assumptions.
Arithmetic mean	Also known as the arithmetic average or simply as the mean or average. The sum of the observations divided by the number of observations. Can be deceptively large when the distribution is skewed by a few very large observations as in a distribution of incomes or body weights. The *median* should be reported in such cases.
Chi-square distribution	A distribution based on theoretical considerations for the square of a normally distributed random variable.
Chi-square statistic	A test statistic based on both the observed values in a contingency table and the values one would expect if the *null hypothesis* were true. With tens of thousands of observations, the chi-square statistic will have the *chi-square distribution*. With small samples, it may have a quite different distribution.
Confidence limits	The boundary values of a confidence interval.
Critical value	The value of a test statistic that separates the values for which we would reject the hypothesis from the values for which we would accept it.
Exact test	The calculated *p-value* of the test is exactly the probability of a *Type I error*; it is not an approximation.
Logistic regression	A statistical method applied to time-to-event data. Applicable even when observations are censored. Used both to extrapolate into the future and to make treatment comparisons.
Median	The 50th percentile. Half the observations are larger than the median, and half are smaller. The *arithmetic mean* and the median of a *normal distribution* are the same.
Minimum relevant differenc	The smallest difference that is of clinical significance.
Normal distribution	A symmetric distribution of values that takes a bell-shaped form. Most errors in observation follow a normal distribution.

Null hypothesis	The hypothesis that there are no (or null) differences in the populations being compared.
Permutation tests	A family of statistical techniques using a variety of test statistics. The *p-values* obtained from these tests are always exact, not approximations.
***p*-Value**	The probability of observing by chance alone a value of the statistic more extreme than the observed value.
Rank tests	The ranks of the observations are used in place of their original values to diminish the effects of extreme observations.
Significance level	Probability of making a *Type I error*. Same as *p-value*.
Student's *t*	See *t-test*.
***t*-Test**	A technique utilizing the *Student's* statistic for comparing the means of two samples.
Type I error	Attributing a purely chance effect to some other cause.
Type II error	Attributing a real effect to chance.
Wilcoxon test	Like the *t-test*, compares the means of two samples, but uses ranks rather than the original observations.

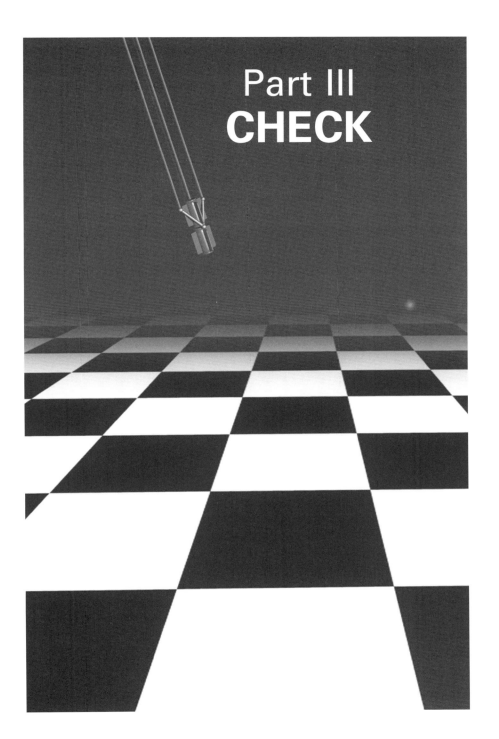

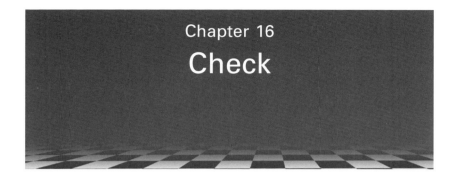

Chapter 16
Check

YOU MAY HAVE TURNED in your report to the regulatory agency. They may even have granted the approval you desired. But unless your company plans on going out of business tomorrow, you still have six important issues to resolve.

1. How will you bring closure to the trials—parting with patients, archiving the data, and publishing the results?
2. What did the trials really cost? Were there avoidable delays?
3. What have you learned during the investigation that would guide in you in expanding or narrowing your original claim?
4. Are there potential adverse effects that warrant further investigation?
5. What have you learned about other diseases and devices or medications that might be of interest to your company?
6. What have you learned that would help you to conduct more effective studies in the future?

CLOSURE

Trial closure has three important aspects: providing for follow-up patient care, making arrangements for storing the data, and arranging for publication of the results.

Patient Care

A patient cannot be discharged from the study until arrangements have been made for continued medical care either from the patient's

---

A Manager's Guide to the Design and Conduct of Clinical Trials, by Phillip I. Good
Copyright ©2006 John Wiley & Sons, Inc.

regular physician (at the patient's expense) or from the appropriate public agency.

If the new treatment represents a demonstrated improvement over existing methodologies, continued supplies must be made available to the patient at no cost until marketing approval is obtained from the regulatory agency.

If the treatment require a tapering-off phase (as do beta-blockers, for example), then supplies must be made available to the each patient until a transition to an alternate treatment is complete.[51]

Data

The original case report forms should be stored in a readily retrievable form (an e-Sub will automatically fill this need). Copies of the master database should be kept both on and off site, at least initially. With the examples of diethylstilbesterol and silicon implants before us, and an increasingly litigious society, it is best to plan on an indefinite storage period for at least one of the copies.

Maintaining archives for samples, X rays, angiograms, and analog EKG and EEG traces can be somewhat more challenging but is also essential. See Bell, Curb, Friedman et al. (1985).

Spreading The News

Klimt and Canner (1979) recommend that in disclosing the results of the trials you follow this sequence: investigators, participants and their physicians, the scientific press, marketing materials. All publications should adhere to CONSORT guideline as described in Chapter 8 and at *http://www.consort-statement.org/*. See also the AMA *Manual of Style* (1994), Bailar and Mosteller (1988), and Long and Secic (1997).

POSTMARKET SURVEILLANCE

Ours is a litigious society. You want to remain aware of any adverse events that could be attributed—rightly or wrongly—to your product or process. Designate an individual (or department) to handle post-market review; provide them with an 800 number and email address. Encourage physicians to report all unanticipated responses to your product, favorable or unfavorable, to this individual. Pay particular attention to adverse events that come to light during your post-trial review.

---

[51]See, for example, Bell, Curb, Friedman et al. (1985).

BUDGET

Considering that pharmaceutical and device firms, large or small, are by definition profit-making concerns, it is amazing how few (none in my experience) ever bother to complete a posttrial review of the trial budget. Alas, those who do not learn from the lessons of history will be forced to repeat them. You cannot control costs or spend your money efficiently until you know what your expenses are.

Your primary objective is to determine the cost of the trials on a per patient basis. Your secondary objectives are to determine the impact of any actual and potential cost cutting.

The cost per patient can be divided into variable and fixed costs. Variable costs include costs of hospitalization (if any), physician visits, drugs and devices, special procedures (angiograms, EKGs) and any other miscellaneous costs *that can be attributed to* a specific patient.

Fixed costs include work-hours invested by you and your staff on all phases of the trials, computer hardware and software, travel, and all other costs that cannot be attributed to patients whose results were used to determine the effectiveness of treatment.

In other words, any costs associated with patients who were interviewed but declared ineligible, who dropped out along the way, and whose records are incomplete contribute only to fixed costs.

CONTROLLING EXPENDITURES

You knew at the start that the most effective way to control costs (apart from the switch from printed forms to electronic data capture) was to hire the right investigators and closely monitor their efforts, and to recruit only those patients who would make a positive contribution to the trials. Of course, this goal is seldom achieved. Now is the time to document anything you have learned during the trials that will help you come closer to this goal on the next go around.

Hopefully, you have kept track of *every* aspect of the trials:

- **Were supplies of drugs/devices/biologics, forms, and sample collection kits always on hand when needed?**
- **Were computers in physician's offices and the associated communication links always in good working order? How quickly were repairs made?**

Inevitably, at one or more points during a set of lengthy trials, a decision is made to trim costs. Not infrequently, the decision is external to the trials themselves, a corporate-level decision, but you as a middle manager had no choice but to go along. Did you make cuts in the appropriate places? What costs ought you to have trimmed instead?

If you'd had more money to spend, how would you have spent it?

PROCESS REVIEW COMMITTEE

The purpose of an after action review is to provide guidance for the conduct of future trials. Were there delays? Redundant or unnecessary efforts or expenses? Could the work have been done more efficiently or effectively?

Strictly speaking, a separate committee ought to be formed to review all nonmedical aspects of the trials including expenditures, workplace efficiency, software development and implementation, manual preparation and quality, training, data management, data integrity, data access, and data security, as well as monitoring costs, methods, and effectiveness. More often the burden of preparing such a report will fall on a single individual. The problem with such a resolution is that no one will read the subsequent report. Consequently, although a single individual, the project leader for example, may be charged with the report preparation, the final result should bear the signatures of all team leaders as well as those of several levels of upper management.

TRIAL REVIEW COMMITTEE

The majority of the remaining issues are best resolved with the aid of a posttrial committee or committees. Membership should include all the original members of the design committee if available, a biostatistician, representatives from the implementation team (which representatives will depend on the issues that have arisen during the trials), all the investigators, one or more members of the safety committee, and representatives of all other project teams in your company.

I'd recommend that the members of the design team, the CRMs, and medical monitor meet separately with the investigators.

INVESTIGATORY DRUG OR DEVICE

The questions to ask will depend on whether the new treatment proved to be a success or a failure and whether the trials themselves were conclusive.

When the treatment is a success, you need to ask:

- **Was the treatment was more effective with some groups of patients than with others?**
- **Were interactions with other treatments uncovered?**
- **Are there other groups of patients and other indications to which the trials could be extended?**

When the treatment is a success, it is not difficult to obtain suggestions for a second set of trials involving a new category of patients or a new indication. But when the treatment is a failure, it is sometimes difficult to find anyone after the trials are over who is knowledgeable enough to suggest a cause. As a new treatment's inadequacies become evident, people leave a project, are reassigned or find reasons for leaving. An immediate postmortem of the trial findings is even more important in such circumstances.

Sometimes the reason for failure is evident. A rare but serious side effect was brought to light. Sometimes it can be more subtle: Too small a starting sample accompanied by a larger than anticipated number of withdrawals led to an inconclusive finish.

Often the principal reasons for failure are those that should have discouraged the trials launch in the first place: Too little was known about the mode of action, about possible interactions with other commonly prescribed treatments. A surgical procedure still was evolving and consequently took on a dozen different forms in the hands of the various investigators.

A treatment can sometimes appear to be a failure solely because the results were inconclusive. Sufficient patients were not enrolled in the trials, and, to the point, too few patients remained after correcting for dropouts, treatment withdrawals, and missing observations.

It is important under these circumstances to recompute the power of test using one of the same computer programs that was used to determine sample size.[52] Excessively low power suggests that additional trials might be called for. See Barnard (1990) and Young, Bresnitz, and Strom (1983).

The reasons underlying excessive numbers of withdrawals and dropouts should be investigated. The treatment regimen should undergo a detailed critical examination. (Was the dose too high or too low? Was the treatment regimen so complex as to preclude adherence?)

Whatever the outcome of the trials, additional consideration may need to be given to secondary responses, interactions, and adverse events.

---

[52]See Chapter 6 and the Appendix.

Detection of secondary beneficial responses that were unanticipated during the design stage (for example, a sedative or an antifebrile effect in addition to an anti-inflammatory) can often be gleaned from the anecdotal accounts of investigators. This is a major reason for including all the investigators in the trial postmortem.

Such accounts may suggest a basis for future trials or for future pre-clinical investigation.

Interactions

Breaking down the data into subsets (female patients, patients with ostial lesions) and analyzing each subset separately often reveals both those patients who are most likely to benefit from the treatment as well as those who are least likely. A new treatment that is at first judged to be unsuccessful may actually prove to have demonstrated potential in specific groups of patients.

Subgroup analyses may also suggest new subsets of covariates to use in patient selection and in baseline adjustment.

Adverse Events

Adverse effects of treatment may remain undetected during clinical trials for at least three reasons:

1. **Restricted set of participants**
2. **Limited follow-up**
3. **Inadequate sample size (particularly for relatively rare side effects)**

Your eligibility criteria may have limited the original trials to males under sixty not suffering from collateral conditions. But physicians are always tempted to extend the range of application of a successful treatment regardless of what it might say on the package insert. To avoid potential litigation, you should consider engaging in follow-up clinical trials that would focus on individuals who were excluded from the original study.

Additional, long-term monitoring of at least a subset of those patients for which you already have such a great store of data is recommended. It offers a way of discovering both 1) additional beneficial effects and 2) delayed adverse effects (thus avoiding or minimizing the impact of subsequent litigation).

Postmarketing analysis typically is based solely on anecdotal accounts. Systematic follow-up has a far greater probability of early detection and of countering false claims.

> **PROJECT WISE, CORPORATION STUPID**
>
> Bumbling Pharmaceuticals had a well-established market share for its A device, but was hoping that E, its new experimental device, might give it total market dominance. Alas, an initial analysis of the data showed that E offered no particular advantage over A. Probing deeper, it was found that when abixcimab, an adjunct given some of the patients, was taken into account, patients without the adjunct did do better with E in some cases. Abixcimab helped patients implanted with the traditional device A, but only worsened their condition when used in conjunction with E.
>
> A further analysis on the basis of sex revealed that although almost 50% of the women given the adjunct along with the experimental procedure suffered a relapse, the standard procedure given in conjunction with abixcimab was 100% effective.
>
> One could visualize the headline, "Bumbling Device 100% effective in women when used in accordance with doctor's instructions," and the resultant improvement in Bumbling's bottom line. But then, I was thinking from the corporation's point of view. In the end, the marketing representative decreed we would just report the combined results. "Our job," she said, "is only to report on the new device."

For example, although many cholesterol-lowering drugs are now on the market, as of this writing only one had sufficient carefully monitored posttrial experience that its manufacturers were permitted to make the claim that it reduced coronary mortality. Naturally, this drug now has the largest market share. And, because I have an adverse reaction to the drug in question—my physician's and my first choice—I can only hope my present lipid-lowering drug ultimately will prove equally effective.

Note: In most countries, you will need to obtain permission from patients to continue surveillance after the scheduled end of the trials.

COLLATERAL STUDIES

I cannot stress sufficiently the importance of including representatives of all study teams, past and present, on posttrial committees.

Every trial results in the uncovering of information that may prove of value in collateral studies or suggests additional applications for existing products. Vice versa, a phenomena that was not well understood in your own trials, and may have proved a barrier to their effective completion, may already have been encountered and overcome by another study team.

Many companies today allow employees to pursue MBAs or doctorates on company time. Yet nothing could be more valuable to an employee and less costly than the shared experiences of other employees.

FUTURE STUDIES
As an aid to future investigations you need to answer and document your answers to all of the following questions:
Data
- Were essential baseline variables and risk factors neglected?
- Were there baseline imbalances? How could they have been prevented?
- Was blinding maintained? If not, why not?
- Did you gather all the information you needed? What other observations should you have recorded? Should alternative measuring techniques have been used?
- Did you gather redundant information? What information should have been omitted? Would there be associated cost savings?

Patients
- Which recruiting strategies were the most effective?
- What was the time course of recruitment?
- How could the ratio of eligible to ineligible patients be increased?
- Were some sites more effective at retaining patients (minimizing withdrawals) than others? Why were they successful?
- Which investigators should be asked to participate in future trials?

In short, the function of posttrial review is to elicit and document anything and everything that might be of assistance to you and your coworkers in future efforts. See also Beck (1996).

FOR FURTHER INFORMATION
American Medical Association. (1994) *Manual of Style* Chicago: AMA.

Bailar JC III; Mosteller F. (1988) Guidelines for statistical reporting for articles in medical journals. Amplifications and explanations. *Ann Intern Med* 108:266–273.

Barnard GA. (1990) Must clinical trials be large? The interpretation of p-values and the combination of test results. *Statist Med* 9:601–614.

Beck B. (1996) *Clinical Trials : Decision Tools For Measuring And Improving Performance*. Buffalo Grove, IL: Interpharm.

Bell RL; Curb JD; Friedman LM et al. (1985) Termination of clinical trials: beta-blocker heart attack trial and the hypertension detection and follow-up program experiences. *Control Clin Trials* 6:102–111.

Klimt CR; Canner PL. (1979) Terminating a long-term clinical trial. *Clin Pharmacol Ther* 25:641–646.

Long TA; Secic M. (1997) *How to Report Statistics in Medicine.* Philadelphia: American College of Physicians.

Schultz KF; Chalmers I; Grimes DA; Altman DG. (1994) Assessing the quality of randomization from reports of controlled trials published in journals of obstetrics and gynecology. *JAMA* 272:125–128.

Schultz KF; Chalmers I; Hayes RJ; Altman DG. (1995) Empirical evidence of bias. Dimensions of methodological quality associates with estimates of treatment effects in controlled trials. *JAMA* 273:408–142.

Young MJ; Bresnitz EA; Strom BI. (1983). Sample size nomograms for interpreting negative clinical studies. *Ann Intern Med* 99:248–251.

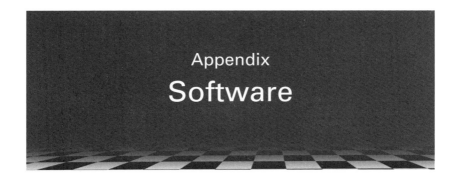

Appendix: Software

> Let the software determine your hardware.
> Good (1984)

An extremely wide choice of software is available to ease your task of designing, managing, and analyzing clinical trials. Some programs offer to do it all, whereas others, more specialized, provide for speech recognition and collecting information from handheld devices.

You will need at least five types of programs; whether you buy them separately or in a comprehensive integrated package is up to you.

1. Project management
2. Data entry
3. Data management
4. Data analysis
5. Utilities

CHOICES

All in One

TrialXS. Fully integrates trial management, electronic data capture, and data management into a single environment. Trial XS/TMS. ClinSource NV, Mechelsesteenweg 455 Bus 2, B-1950 Kraainem, Belgium. +32 (0)2 766 00 80. *info@clinsource.com.*

A Manager's Guide to the Design and Conduct of Clinical Trials, by Phillip I. Good
Copyright ©2006 John Wiley & Sons, Inc.

Oracle Clinical. Has the standard features of Oracle. Automatically create views corresponding to each case report form (CRF) and automatically extracts data into SAS for analysis. It's easy to create custom views combining data from multiple CRFs, to query the data online, and to create any number of data snapshots for interim analysis during normal data processing.

Provides your staff with the ability to visualize the planned, projected, and actual patient enrollment and study timelines, develop detailed visit schedule specification and tracking, including the identification of missing and late (CRFs), manage and track treatment blind breaks, and track patient availability and withdrawal information.

On the downside, Oracle Clinical is less flexible than Oracle, and we've found it easier to create reports and CRF's in the original, less expensive product. Oracle Corporation, 1-888-672-2534.

MetaTrial System. VIPS., One West Pennsylvania Avenue, Baltimore, MD 21204, 410-832-8300.

Almost All in One

SAS. SAS afficinados swear that with all modules in place, SAS can be used to build e-CRFs, manage the data, and perform the analyses. We're not one, so we've listed SAS below under "Data Analysis."

Clindex. Data entry, data management, and payment management. Easy-to-build screens can be generated directly from any word processor document. Then add edit checks and data validation, radio buttons and drop-down menus. Built around the Sybase InfoMaker® screen and report painter and Sybase SQL Anywhere® database, it provides an easy-to-use SQL environment. Double clicking on a patient or CRF in any report can be used to display all that patient's CRFs in read-only or update mode. Fortress Medical Systems, Inc., 901 1st St North, Hopkins, MN 55343. 952.238-9010. *info@fortressmedical.com.*

Project Management

TrialWorks^{TM}. Tracks your project management data by study and by site. Multiple users can simultaneously access all your tracking data. Tracking is comprehensive and includes IRB approvals, 1572s, patient enrollment and withdrawals, regulatory submissions, and investigator, vendor, and CRA payments. TrialWorks then uses that data to produce over 100 reports. ClinPhone, 7 Rozel Road, Princeton NJ 08540, *www.trialtrac.com*.

PharmaTrack™. A Web based study tracking system to track clinical trial progress for management. Site plans track critical tasks and milestones you define for each participating investigator, such as site initiation or enrollment period. Patient progress can be similarly tracked, either at a site summary level such as Total Enrolled or down to patient-specific items such as Signed Informed Consent or Visit 3 Completed. Cintelligence from the same vendor lets you track performancew across products. Not only can you track study progress and on-time performance from concept to completion, but you can monitor staff effectness and investigator timeless and quality across multiple projects and can use past performance to help you milestone future studies. **3C:** 93 Cutler Road, Greenwich, CT 06831. 310-312-9516. *http://www.3cpharma.com/products.asp*.

DATA ENTRY

Handheld Devices

Gather information from the patient's bedside or have the patient himself record the exact time and date medication was taken or symptoms observed.

Touch Screen

HCOL Clinical Study. Includes electronic touch screen and web interfaces for many commonly used patient questionnaires. Spinal Outcomes Lumbar (SOL), Spinal Outcomes Cervical (SOC), Electronic Pain Diagram, Visual Analog Scale (VAS), Medical History Questionnaire, SF-36, the Oswestry Disability Questionnaire, Neck Disability Index, Johns Hopkins Cervical and Lumbar Outcomes Questionnaires, Others . . . *http://www.hcol.com/*

Speech Recognition

PocketTrials. Uses structured speech recognition to make it easy to enter data in hands-busy environments. Support is catch as catch can. 301-776-1196. *support@PocketTrials.com*.

e-CRFs

When evaluating products in this category, look for the following essentials:

- Range and logic validation checks
- Pull-down selection menus
- Radio buttons and toggle buttons

Do It Yourself

StudyBuilder. Even if you decide to buy another, more expensive product, StudyBuilder is the ideal way to introduce your CRMs and medical staff to computerized case report forms. The system utilizes a point and click method that allows you to build a form by dragging questions out of their extensive built-in library of validated study questions, and dropping them into place. Fields are validated, and pop-up warning messages appear on the screen if bounds are exceeded.

Build the form in a language with which your staff is familiar, then have it immediately translated into Dutch, English, French, German, Italian, Spanish, Modern Standard Arabic, or Japanese for use in other countries. Contains built-in support for downloading data onto PCs via serial, infrared and USB ports on many platforms including the web! 268 Bush Street, Suite 1123, San Francisco CA 94104, 1 800 727 2304 *US@STUDYBUILDER.COM*; Postbus 177, 1000 Ad Amsterdam, The Netherlands, +31 (71) 514 2988, *NL@STUDYBUILDER.COM*; Level 11 Park West Building, 6-12-1 Nishi-Shinjuku, Shinjuku-Ku Tokyo, 160-0023 Japan, *JP@STUDYBUILDER.COM*.

Sybase InfoMaker®. Screen and report painter lets you build the most user-friendly forms. Requires sophisticated programmers. Accepts PowerBuilder input. For Windows, UNIX or LINUX. Sybase, One Sybase Drive Dublin, CA 94568. 1-800-8SYBASE.

Data Collection Via the Web

Clinical Discovery Platform. Simplified Clinical Data Systems, 12 Middle Street, Amherst, NH 03031. (603) 673-1900. http://www.simplifiedclinical.com/

Clintrinet. Each trial is assigned a website that becomes the central workplace for all trial personnel and warehouse for all trial data and records. Data entry includes range and logic checks. ClinicalTrialsNet Inc, 12 John Street, Charleston, SC 29403, 843.965.5598, *info@clinicaltrialsnet.com.*

***Datatrak EDC*™**. 6150 ParklandBlvd., Mayfield Heights, Ohio 44124, 440-443-0082 Rochusstrasse 65 D-53121Bonn, Germany, :+49-228-979-8330, *products@datatraknet.com*

Preparing the Common Technical Document

***EZsubs*®**. Include templates for the Common Technical Document and a complete electronic Common Technical Document solution, which may be used immediately to help prepare submissions to the new standards. EZsubs includes Xref Manager, a sophisticated cross-referencing tool, ideally suited for preparing both paper cross-references and the electronic hyperlinks required by electronic submissions and the electronic Common Technical Document. From CDC Solutions, *http://www.electronic-common-technical-document.com/*

FirstDoc R&D. Provides CTD authoring templates in MS Word to help ensure a consistent look and feel of the CTD application. Document inventory capabilities include support for ICH guidelines and CTD/eCTD submission. Open architecture that supports scalability, internationalism, localization and multilingual interfaces. Regulation compliance including electronic signature capabilities, 21 CFR Part 11 compliance for closed and regulates systems, 21 CFR Part 11 audit trail Work process improvements such as CTD authoring templates, autopopulation of document properties, configurable version numbering and workflow review and approval processes. 800-345-0957. *http://www.fcg.com/life-sciences/FirstDoc-Research-and-Development-RD.asp*

DATA MANAGEMENT

When selecting a database management system there are five key areas on which to focus: 1) ease of formulating queries, 2) speed of retrieval of data, 3) ease of updating data, 4) ease of restructuring the database, and 5) ease of integrating other applications including data entry and statistical software.

Oracle. Comprehensive and reliable. If you think like a programmer, then Oracle is remarkably easy to use to create or interrogate a clinical database. For UNIX Oracle Corporation, 1-888-672-2534. http://www.oracle.com/global/index.html?content.html.

Sybase SQL Anywhere. For Windows, UNIX, or LINUX. Sybase, One Sybase Drive Dublin, CA 94568. 1-800-8SYBASE.

C-ISAM. Although not a relational database, you don't have to sift through records to get to the data you want. B+ tree index architecture makes data retrieval fast and easy. C-ISAM uses index entries as keys that point to records. These keys allow you to find the specific pieces of data you want, without having to look at extra records. On top of that, C-ISAM uses techniques to compress the keys for efficient index storage and processing. The reduced key size means faster response and better performance for the end user. For UNIX. IBM.

DATA ENTRY AND DATA MANAGEMENT

Small-Scale Clinical Studies

Microsoft Access. Choice of spreadsheet entry or more sophisticated forms. Provides toggle buttons but no pull-down menus. Includes range and logic checks. PC-based and can be purchased from virtually any computer or office supply outlet.

Advanced Revelation/OpenInsight. Excellent data manager with minimal memory requirements. Flexible data entry including pull-down menus, range and logic checks. Revelation Software 800/262-4747, +44 (0) 1908 233255, +61-2-9939-6399. *info@revelation.com*.

Clinical Database Managers

The members of this extensive class are both expensive and generally unsatisfactory because they force you to adapt your study to their software, thus violating the first rule of trial design to let your reports determine the data to be collected.

Acceliant^{TM}. Includes a medical image management module. Megasoft, 85, Kutchery Road, Millennium Center, Mylapore Chennai-600 004 +91-44-24616768. *lifesciences@megasoft.com*

Clintrial. This product has seen unsettling times during a period of mergers and acquisitions, but emerged looking better than ever. Provides CDISC support and can be integrated with their electronic data capture and drug safety monitoring software. Phase Forward Incorporated, 880 Winter Street, Waltham, MA 02451-1623 +1 888 703 1122. http://www.phaseforward.com/products_cdms_clintrial.html

SyMetric. SyMetric Sciences, Inc. 1-2082 Sherbrooke West, Montreal, Quebec. Canada H3H 1G5. Major@SyMetric.ca. http://www.symetric.ca/

DATA ANALYSIS

SAS. Overpriced, cumbersome, and unevenly documented. Large number of statistical routines with many options for table creation and graphs. Too few built-in nonparametric routines, but the statistical literature is filled with SAS macros for a wide variety of supplemental procedures including bootstrap and density estimates. Knowledgeable programmers are essential but widely available.

Thoroughly validated and has been used in hundreds of submissions. SAS Institute Inc., SAS Campus Drive, Cary, NC 27513. (Windows, MVS, CMS, VMS, Unix). *www.sas.com*.

SPSS. The poor man's SAS, offers ease of use along with a large number of statistics. A bootstrap subcommand provides bootstrap estimates of standard errors and confidence limits. Thoroughly validated and has been used in dozens of submissions. (Windows). SPSS Inc., 444 North Michigan Avenue, Chicago, Illinois 60611. 312/329-2400. *www.spss.com*.

Stata. Provides a comprehensive set of statistics routines plus subroutines and preprogrammed macros for bootstrap, density estimation, and permutation tests. Programmable with many flexible grapics routines. (Windows, Unix) Stata Corp, 702 University Drive East, College Station TX 77840. 800/782-8272. *www.stata.com*.

Data Desk/Activ Stats/DataDesk XL. The best program I know for exploratory data analysis. Windows and Macintosh versions *info@datadesk.com http://www.datadesk.com/DataDesk/system.shtml*

StatXact. While not a comprehensive statistics package, it is a must for the exact analysis of contingency tables (categorical or ordered data) and should be purchased along with one of the four statistics programs listed above. The StatXact manual is a textbook in its own right. The program is thoroughly validated and has been used in dozens of submissions. Versions for Windows or Unix. Also available as an add-on module for both SAS and SPSS. Cytel Software Corporation, 675 Massachusetts Avenue, Cambridge, MA 02139. 617-661-2011. *www.cytel.com.*

NPC TEST. The only statistics program on the market today that provides for multi-factor analysis by permutation means. Cutting edge, but has yet to be validated. A demonstration version, SAS macro, and S-Plus code may be downloaded from *http://www.stat.unipd.it/~pesarin/software.html.*

UTILITIES

Sample Size Determination

Power and Precision. This menu-driven program can be used to determine fixed sample size for tests of proportions (including equivalence), means, RxC contingency tables, analysis of variance, regression, and survival analysis. **Biostat**, 14 North Dean Street, Englewood, NJ 07631 USA, (201) 541-5688, *www.power-analysis.com.*

PASS 2000. Lets you solve for power, sample size, effect size, and alpha level and automatically creates appropriate tables and charts of the results. Covers an extremely wide range of statistical procedures including Fisher's exact test, the Wilcoxon test, factorials, and repeated measures. 490-page manual contains tutorials, examples, annotated output, references, formulas, verification, and complete instructions on each procedure. NCSS Statistical Software, 329 North 1000 East, Kaysville, Utah 84037. (800) 898-6109 Download free demo version from *http://www.ncss.com.*

nQuery Advisor. Helps you determine sample size for 50+ design and analysis combinations. Windows. Statistical Solutions, 8 South Bank, Crosse's Green, Cork, Ireland. 800/262-1171. +353 21 4319629. *www.statsol.ie.*

S+SeqTrial. An extra-cost module for S-PLUS, yields sequential designs for clinical trials. 800.569.0123 *http://www.insightful.com/products/seqtrial/features.asp.*

Screen Capture

Winrunner. Mercury Interactive, 1325 Borregas Avenue, Sunnyvale, CA 94089. 1-800-TEST-911, +33 1 40 83 68 68, *Info-France@mercury-eur.com*.

Silktest. Segue Software, 201 Spring St, Lexington, MA 02421. 800.287.1329 For other offices, see *http://www.segue.com/about-segue/offices.asp* or *contact info@segue.com*.

Data Conversion

DBMS Copy. Lets you exchange files among two dozen statistics packages, a dozen plus data base managers, and multiple versions of a half dozen spreadsheets. UNIX and Windows versions. DataFlux Corporation, 4001 Weston Parkway Suite 300, Cary, NC 27513, (877) 846-3589, +44 (0)1753 868 725. *sales@dataflux.com*.

Author Index

Abrams, J., 53, 120
Abramson, N. S., 219
Adams, J. R., 73
Ader, H. J., 74
Agras, W. S., 118
Albain, K. S., 53
Altman, D. G., 204, 219, 235
American Medical Association, 234
Anderson. W., 208
Angell, M., 4, 58,
Applegate, W. B., 119
Armitage, P., 185, 187
Arriaza, E., 158
Artinian, N. T., 188
Asilomar Working Group on Recommendations for Reporting Clinical Trials in the Biomedical Literature, 105
Ayala, E., 179, 188

Backhouse, M. E., 73
Bailar, J. C., 219, 228, 234
Baker, A., 119
Baltch, A. L., 115, 120
Barbui, C., 57
Barkhof, F., 74
Barnard, G. A., 231, 234
Baron, J., 120
Barr, R. G., 118, 120

Barsky, A. J., 119, 188
Bassion, S., 141
Beck, B., 234
Begg, C. B., 105, 219
Bell, R. L., 228, 234
Benjamin, H. H., 213, 220
Benedetti, J., 51
Bennett, C. L., 73
Berger, V., 60, 179, 188, 198, 219
Berlin, J. A., 73
Beveridge, R. A., 53
Birnbaum, Y., 51
Blair, R. C., 221
Blaskowski, T. P., 119
Bluman, L. G., 120
Bolanos, E., 158
Booth, A., 52
Bradford, R. H., 118
Brandt, C. A., 155, 158
Brawley, O., 53, 120
Breen, N., 53, 120
Brennan, A., 52
Bresnitz, E. A., 231, 235
Bristol, H., 158
Butow, P. N., 119
Butte, A. J., 121
Byar, D. P., 220

Campbell, M., 73–74
Canner, P. L., 228, 235

Cantor, A., 73
Carey, T. S., 108, 119
Cassileth, B., 74
CAST (Cardiac Arrhythmia Suppression Trial), 40, 52
Cavan, B. N., 73
Celano, P., 73
Chadwick, B., 119
Chalmers, I., 235
Chalmers, T. C., 61, 73
Cheng, S. C., 74
Chernick, M., 36
Chilcott, J. F., 30, 33
Cho, M., 105
Chow, S.-C., 51
Christian, M. C., 53, 120
Chuang-Stein, C., 219
Ciudad, A., 158
Claxton, K., 73
Cleveland, W. S., 219
Cocchetto, D. M., 51
Coglianese, M. E., 119
Coltman, C. A., Jr., 53
Conlon, M., 158
Conover, W., 209, 219
Conway, M. D., 51
Collins, J. F., 30, 33
Coyle, C., 120
Cramer, J. A., 119, 120
Crowley, J., 51, 53

A Manager's Guide to the Design and Conduct of Clinical Trials, by Phillip I. Good
Copyright ©2006 John Wiley & Sons, Inc.

Curb, J. D., 113, 120, 228, 234
Curtis, R. C., 119

Dafra, P., 219
Dar, R., 219
Date, C. J., 158
Davis, C. E., 117, 119
DeMets, D. L., 47, 112, 117, 120, 185, 188
Desmond, J., 52
Djulbegovic, B., 57
Dmitrienko, A., 219
Donegani, M., 219
Donovan, J. L., 119
Dore, C. J., 204, 219
Dowsett, S. M., 119

Eastwood, S., 105
Ebi, O., 52
Ederer, R., 61, 73
Egin, D., 33
Ellis, P. M., 113, 120
Elwood, J. M., 73
Entsuah, A. R., 220
Ernst, E., 74
Evans, M., 117, 119
Expert Working Group (Efficacy) of the International Conference on Harmonisation of Technical Requirements for Registration of Pharmaceuticals for Human Use (ICH), See also ICH, 106
Exner, D. V., 60

Favalli, G., 49
Fay, M. P., 221
Fayers, P., 51
Fazzari, M., 36, 52
Feinstein, A. R., 49, 117, 119, 220
Fernandez, G., 155, 159
Fields, K. K., 73
Fienberg, S. E., 220
Fleisher, G. R., 121
Fleming, T. R., 40, 47, 188
Foote, M., 106
Ford, L., 53

Francis, Q., 208, 220
Freedman, L., 12, 212, 220
Friedman, L. M., 51, 112, 117, 119, 228, 234
Froelicher, E. S., 188
Furberg, C. D., 51, 112, 117, 119
Fukui, T., 112, 120

Gail, M. H., 220
Gandy, B. G., 157, 158
Garattini, S., 73
Garcia-Molina, H., 158
George, S. L., 52, 221
Gillat, D., 119
Gillum, R. F., 119, 188
Gitanjali, B., 119
Givens, S. V., 106
Goldman, D. P., 51
Good, P. I., 56, 92, 106, 197, 199, 201, 211–216, 220
Gordon, D. J., 119
Gordon, M. E., 118, 120
Grambsch, P. M., 66, 74
Gray, R., 220
Green, S., 51
Greenberg, B., 47
Greene, H. L., 49
Grimes, D. A., 235

Haidich, A. B., 119, 176, 188
Hamdy, F. C., 119
Hampshire, M., 120
Hamrell, M. R., 188
Handberg-Thurmond, E., 115, 119
Harrington, D., 52
Harris, R. J., 119
Hayes, R., 51
Hayes, R. J., 235
Haynes, R. B., 115, 119
Heller, G., 36, 52
Herman, A. A., 53
Hesen, W., 158
Heymer, J., 155, 159
Hibberd, P. L., 121
Hilton. J., 208, 220
Hochberg, A., 180–183
Holborow, D. W., 120
Horney, A., 33

Horton, R., 105
Howard, M., 220
Howell, C. L., 33
Hudson, C., 120
Hujoel, P. P., 120
Hunninghake, D. B., 119
Hutchins, L. F., 45, 53

Iber, F. L., 51
International Committee of Medical Journal Editors, 106
International Study of Infarct Survival Collaborative Group, 214, 220
Ioannidis, J. P., 119, 176, 188
Ivanova, A., 185, 188, 198, 219

Jones, B., 73

Kaplan, R., 53, 120
Karnon, J., 52
Karras, B. T., 158
Katz, R. J., 49
Keith, S. J., 45, 53, 119
Kelly, M. A., 158
Kelsey, S. F., 219
Kent, E., 33
Kenward, M. G., 73
Kertes, P. J., 51
Kessler, D. A., 106
Keyserling, T., 119
Kinsinger, L., 119
Kirk, G., 33
Klimt, C. R., 228, 235
Kloner, R. A., 51
Knipschild, P., 117, 119
Krishnen, A., 207, 221
Kuderer, N. M., 73

Lacevic, M., 73
Lachin, J. M., 185, 188, 220
Lallas, C. D., 155, 158
Lan, G., 185, 188
Lane, J. A., 119
Lang, J. M., 117, 120, 203, 206, 220
Larus, J., 140
Laska, E. M., 52

Leffers, P., 117, 119
Leveillee. R. J., 158
Lin, D. Y., 185, 188
Lingeman, J. E., 158
Linnet, K., 214, 220
Liu, J.-P., 51
Liuni, C., 33
Lock, S. P., 111, 120
Long, T. A., 106, 228, 235
Lopez-Carrero, C., 155, 158
LRC Investigators, 41, 53
Lu, C., 158
Lung Health Study Research Group, 120
Lunneborg, C., 199
Lyman, G. H., 73

MacKay, R. J., 217, 220
MacKillop, N., 179, 188
Manly, B. F. J., 208, 220
Marenco, L., 158
Margitic, S., 115, 120
Marks, R., 155, 158
Marquez, L. O., 141
Marshall, G. D., 118
Martin, S., 33
Maschio, G., 53
Massoth, K. M., 120
Matthews, J. N. S., 74
Matts, J. P., 188
Mattson, M. E., 113, 120
Max, M. B., 52
McArdle, R., 113, 120
McBride, P. E., 108, 120
McCabe, M., 53
McCormick, M., 119
McInnes, P. M., 52
McSherry, F., 33
Mehta, C. R., 185, 188, 220
Mendes, A., 157, 158
Metz, J. M., 120
Migrino, R. Q., 53
Milgrom, P. M., 117, 120
Miller, D. H., 74
Moher, D., 105
Moke, P., 221
Molenbergs, G., 219
Moore, T., 49, 53, 56
Morita, S., 112, 120
Moseley, J. B., 58

Mosteller, F., 219, 228, 234
Moye, L. A., 49, 53, 214, 220
Mulay, M., 51
Municio, M., 158
Murray, P. J., 51

Nadkarni, P., 158
Nardi, R. V., 51
National Cancer Institute, 52
Neal, D. E., 119
Ness, R. B., 73
Nielsen, O. S., 141
Noble, S., 119

O'Brien, P., 208, 220
Ockene, J. K., 115, 120
O'Connor, M., 106
Offen, W., 219
Oldford, R. W., 217, 220
Oldham, J., 158
Oldrizzi, L., 53
Oliver, S. E., 119
Oikin, I., 105
Omer, H., 219
Oosterhoff, J., 220

Pablos-Mendez, A., 118, 120
Pajak, T., 52
Pandian, D. G., 119
Paoletti, L. Q., 52
Park, T. S., 188
Parker, B., 120
Patel, N. R., 188, 197, 220
Paul, J., 158
Pearle, M. S., 158
Pearson, R., 181–183
Pecorelli, S., 52
Peddiwell, J. A., 213, 221
Pepine, C. J., 158
Permutt, T., 198, 219
Pesarin, F., 185, 188, 208, 220
Peters, T. J., 119
Peterson, B. L., 221
Piantadosi, S., 74, 220
Pitt, B., 52
Pledger, G. W., 206, 220
Pocock, S., 52
Portenoy, R. K., 52

Posnett, J., 73
Pothoff, R. F., 221
Preminger, G. M., 158
Prescott, T., 158
Prien, R. F., 52
Prokscha, S., 159

Rahman, M., 112, 120
Ramos, J., 158
Raveendran, R., 119
Redmond, C., 52
Regan, K., 120
Renard, J., 52
Resio, M. A., 115, 120
Rifkin, R. M., 53
Riley, W. A., 51
Robinson, D. S., 52
Roden, D. M., 49, 52
Rondel, R. K., 159
Rosenberger, W. P., 185, 188
Ruffin, M. T., 120
Rumsey, D., 221
Rush, H., 118, 121
Rutman, O., 106

Sackett, D. L., 115, 119
Sacks, H. S., 61, 74
Sakamoto, J., 112, 120
Salsburg, D. S., 199, 208–209, 219, 221
Sateren, W. B., 45, 53, 113, 120
Schacter, L., 158
Schechtman, K. B., 118, 120
Scher, H. I., 36, 52
Schildkraut, J., 120
Schron, E. B., 115, 120
Schultz, K. F., 235
Schumaker, S. A., 115, 120
Schwope, J. P., 158
Secic, M., 106, 203, 206, 220, 228, 235
Seib, R., 158
Senchaudhuri, P., 188
Serlin, A., 219
Shea, S., 118, 120
Shih, J. H., 185, 188, 221
Shorack, M. A., 113, 120
Shuster. J. J., 68, 74

Siegmund, H., 185, 188
Simon, R., 61, 74
Slud, E., 185, 188
Smith, H., 73
Smith, M., 53, 120
Smith, R. L., 221
Smith, R. P., 115, 119
Smythe, R. T., 188
Spence, E., 33
Spilker, B., 51, 110, 120
Stewart, F. M., 53
Stewart, H., 141
Stinnett, S., 33
Strom, B. I., 231, 235
Sturdee, D. W., 115, 120
Sugarman, J., 114, 120
Sujindra, S., 119
Sutton-Tyrell, K. S., 219
Switula, D., 106
Sylvester, R., 220

Tan, W. Y., 220
Tappenden, P., 52
Tattersall, M. H., 119
Taylor, D. W., 115, 119

Thall, P. R., 74
Therasse, P., 141
Theriault, R. L., 53
Therneau, T. M., 66, 74
Thompson, A. J., 74
Tilley, B. C., 113, 120
Topol, E., 53
Torgerson, D., 73, 74
Trivedi, M. H., 118, 121
Troendle, J. E., 221
Tsiatis, A. A., 197, 220
Tubridy, N., 65, 74

Ullman, J. D., 158
Unger, J. M., 53
Ungerleider, R., 53, 120

van Oosterom, A. T., 141
Vander Wal, J. S., 188
Vantongelen, K., 52
Varley, S. A., 159
Vermorken, J. B., 52
Verweij, J., 141
Vickers, A., 61, 74
Violante, A., 73

Wang, Y., 185, 188
Wears, R. I., 221
Webb, C., 159
Weerahandi, S., 208, 221
Weiand, H. S., 52
Wei, L. J., 47, 185, 188
Weiner, D. L.,121
Weinstein, P., 120
Weiss, R. B., 43
Wells, R., 111
Westfall, D. H., 207, 221
Widom, J., 158
Wieand, H. S., 52
Williams, L. A., 53
Williford, W. D., 30
Willman, D., 11
Woodford, F. P., 106
Wűbbelt, P., 155, 159

Yao, Q., 72, 74
Young, M. J., 231, 235
Young, S. S., 207, 221
Yusef, S., 33

Zelen, M., 204, 221

Subject Index

AAR. See After-action review (AAR)
Abnormal values, 10
Acceliant™ software, 242
Access software, 26
Accuracy, 193–194
Active (positive) controls, 57, 61
Ad hoc hypotheses, 215
Adaptive design, 185
Adjuvant treatment, 196
Advanced Revelation, 242
Adverse events
 forms, 76
 collection, 41, 91
 list, 8, 103
 monitoring, 170
 policy, 179, 232
 reports, 87, 99, 179, 207
Adverse Event Reporting System (AERS), 182
After-action review (AAR), 83, 230
AIDS, 62
AMA Manual of Style, 228
Analysis of variance, 195, 222
Anecdotal studies, 88
Angiograms, 206
Animal experiments, 88

Appointments, missed, 75
Arithmetic mean, 222
Aspirin, 5
Attorney, 28
Audit trail, 132, 145, 157

Baseline
 analysis, 194, 203
 data, 41, 49, 125
 measures, 18, 36, 56
Baxter, 4
Baycol/Lipobay, 4
Behrens-Fisher problem, 208
Bias, 59
Biologics, 18
Binary restenosis,
Binomial data, 202
Blinding, 36, 60–61
Blocking, 56
Blocked randomization,
Blood tests, 40
Bonferroni inequality, 214
Bootstrap, 65, 212
Box and whiskers plot, 193
Breaking the code, 186
Breast implants, 4, 58
Budgets and Expenditures, 50, 118, 141, 186, 229

CANDA. See Computer-aided new drug application (CANDA), 124
Cardiac arrhythmia suppression, 48
Case controls, 71
Case-control studies, 88
Case report forms, 125
 electronic, 130
 storing, 9
Categorical data, 196
Cause and effect relation, 211
CDISC
 guidelines, 125, 133
 Metadata Model, 133
Censored data, 201
Character data
 storing and retrieving, 12
Checklists
 comprehensive, 161
 design, 35, 50, 80
 future studies, 234
 measurements, 42
 preventive measures, 43
Chi-square
 analysis, 222
 distribution, 196, 222
Cholesterol-lowering drugs, 126

A Manager's Guide to the Design and Conduct of Clinical Trials, by Phillip I. Good
Copyright ©2006 John Wiley & Sons, Inc.

C-ISAM, 242
Clinical Discovery
    Platform, 240
Clindex software, 238
Clinical
    review, see AAR
    sites, see Sites
    follow-up, see Follow-up
    investigators, see
        Investigators
Clinical research monitors
    (CRMs), 24, 26, 165
    responsibilities of, 28,
        126, 138–139, 166,
        169–173, 175, 178
Clinical Resource Centers,
    109
Clinical trials
    closure, 46, 72, 227
    cost of, 72
    cut-off dates, 201
    delays, 229
    registry, 107, 113
    single versus multiple,
        36
    termination and
        extension, 184
    time line, 45, 90
Clinical vs statistical
    significance, 217
Clintrial software, 242
Clintrinet software, 240
Closure, 46, 72, 227
Code cracking, 47, 62, 77
Coding systems, 131–132,
    153
Cofactors, 202
Collateral studies, 233
Committees, (see Review
    Committees)
Common Technical
    Document, 37, 83–86
Competing events, 206
Compliance
    increasing, 97
    monitoring, —,
    staff contribution to
Computer-aided new drug
    application
    (CANDA), 104
Computer-assisted data
    entry, 123

Concurrent medications,
    48, 76
Confidence intervals, 191,
    222
Confidentiality, patient,
    155
CONSORT statement,
    105
Contract research
    organizations
    (CROs), 31, 109
Contracts, drafting, 28
Controls, 57
Cost
    considerations, 72
    overruns, 172
    tracking, (see Budgets
        and Expenditures)
CPHS. See Committee for
    the Protection of
    Human Subjects
    (CPHS)
Critical value, 222
Critical terms, 49
CRMs. See Clinical
    research monitors
    (CRMs)
CROs. See Contract
    research
    organizations (CROs)
Crossover design, 70
Crossovers, 205
Cross reactions, 17

Data
    analysis, see Statistical
        analysis
    collecting, 8, 123
    fraudulent, 78
    missing, 178, 205
    monitoring, 78, 180–182
    permanent storage, 228
    repeated tests on, 214
    security, 155
    storage, 133, 156
    transfer, 154
    types of, 64, 190
    visualization, 181
Database management
    systems (DBMS), 150
Database manager, 30,
    156

Database
    access, 148, 155
    backup, 158
    combining, 151
    protection, 157
    regulatory agency access
    types, 143–148
    client-server, 150
    testing, 158
Data Desk/Activ
    Stats/DataDesk XL,
    243
Data entry
    computer-assisted, 10,
        43, 180
    development, 123–131
    via internet, 155
    standardization, 49
    technology, 9
    training for, 139
Data specifications table,
    124
Datatrak EDC™, 241
DB2, 151
DBMS Copy, 245
DBMS. See Database
    management systems
    (DBMS)
Deming regression, 213
Demographics, 103
Design
    checklist, 50
    decisions, 35
    team, 23–25
Documentation
    guidelines for, 83–106
    of software, 218
    checklist, 162
Domain tables, 152
Doses, missed, 75
Dow Corning, 58
Downsizing, 3
Dropouts, 69, 178,
    205

Economic models, 73
e-CRF. See Electronic,
    case report form
    (e-CRF)
EDC. See Electronic, data
    capture
EEG, 29

Efficacy measures, (see Endpoints)
Efficacy trials, 8
Electronic
　case report form (e-CRF), 123
　data capture, 1–3, 132,
　submission (e-Sub), 1, 10
Eligibility
　determination, 45, 112
　requirements, 18, 44, 70, 78, 89, 232
Endpoints, 9
　Reporting, 204
　secondary, 41
　surrogate. 38, 39
Enrollment
　ethical considerations, 114
　monitoring, 77, 176
Equivalence
　demonstrating, 68
　testing for, 209
Error sources, 3, 9–10, 27, 42, 49, 123, 131, 152, 181, 199, 213
Erythromycin, 44
Ethical considerations, 93, 114
Exact test, 222
Exception
　handling, 91
　investigator related, patient related, 103
Expenditures. (see Budgets and Expenditures)
Experimental design, 43, 55
Exponential distribution, 66
External review panels (see Review Committees)
EZsubs®, 241

Facilities, changes in, 171
FDA. See Food and Drug Administration (FDA)
File access, 155

Final reports, 102
First Doc R&D, 241
Fisher's exact test, 92, 196
Flat file database, 143
Follow-up, 45, 125
　missed appointments, 76
　file, 144
　procedures, 91
Food and Drug Administration (FDA), 18, 83, 104, 109, 124, 182, 208
Forecasting models, 176
Formal testing team, 27
Fractional factorial design, 71
Fraudulent data, 78
F-test, 198
Future studies, 233

Gant chart, 26, 125
Globalview operating system, 27
Government regulations, European, 37
Groupings, pre-defined, 126

Handheld devices, 239
Hardware, 27, 229, 162
Hardware checklist, 162
HCOL Clinical Study, 239
Health fairs, 114
Hierarchical databases, 145, 153
Histogram, 181
Historical databases, 71, 107
HTML format, 99–102

ICH guidelines, 38
IHS Guidelines, 203
Implementation team, 19
Ineligible individuals, 69, 205
Informed consent form, 94
Instructions,
　holes in, 48
Intent-to-treat, 19, 63
Interactions (drug), 44, 69, 231

Interest, loss of, 115, 172–174
Interim reports, 83
Investigator
　categories, 167
　manuals, 43
　meetings, 168
　motivators, 110, 173
　payment, 13, 173
　rapport, 167
　relations, 123
　responsibilities, 92
　retention, 111, 173
　recruitment efforts, 28
In vitro/in vivo experiments, 5, 35
ISAM, 149

Journal articles, drafting and publishing, 104, 228

Karnofsky Index, 202
Key fields, 149, 152
Keypunch instructions, 131
Kick-off meetings, 168
KISS, 11, 70, 93
Kruskall-Wallace test, 199

Laboratories
　computerization, 9
　paying, 13
　guidelines, 97
　results validation, 180
Lawsuit, 58
Lead software developer, 125
Lipid-lowering therapies, 44
Logistic regression, 222
Log-rank test, 202
Lung cancer data, 200

Management, 4
Manuals. See Procedures manuals
Manufacturing specialist, 26
Marketing representative, 25
Maximum tolerated dose, 35

SUBJECT INDEX   253

Measurements checklist, 42
Median, 193, 222
Medical monitors, 24, 166, 168, 184, 230
Medication
  adjusting, (see Intent-to-treat)
MeDRA, 86–87
Menus, 129
MetaTrial software, 238
Metoprolol, 39
Metric data, 192, 198
Microsoft Access, 150
Milestones, 25
Minimum effective dose, 35
Minimum relevant difference, 209, 222
Missed appointments, 75
Monitoring, 1, 165
  enrollment, 77
  for quality, 176
  long term, 232
Motrin™, 37, 39
Multicenter trial, 3
Multiple databases, 151
Multiple trials, 36
Multivariate statistical, 186

Network database, 146
New drug applications (NDA), 104
Newsletter, 116, 172
Noncompliant patients, 75, 205
Nonparametric methods, 199
Normal distribution, 65, 222
NPC Test, 244
NQuery Advisor, 244
Null hypothesis, 198, 223

Objectives, 37, 186
Object-oriented databases, 150
O'Brien test, 208
Odds ratio, 191
Open-ended reporting, 123

Oracle software, 26, 150, 238, 241
Oral contraceptives, 44
Ordinal data, 194, 197
Outcome measures, 90
Outcomes, anticipated, 8
Outliers, 199, 206

Paperless system, 1
Parametric methods, 198
Pass 2000, 244
Passive (negative) controls, 57
Patients
  care, 227
  compliance, 97, 116
  confidentiality, 155
  deaths, 171
  follow up, 76, 91
  instructions, 43, 76
  ID, 153
  loss adjustment, 69, 207
  manual, 43
  motivating, 116
  noncompliance, 42
  payment, 95
  population, 4, 36, 44, 107, 114,
  records, 93
  recruitment, 112
  retaining, 115
  selection, 17, 89
  telephone contact, 116
  withdrawals, 63, 91, 103, 165, 178
Payment, advance, 173
Permutation tests, 223, 199
Pfizer, 4
Pharmaceuticals checklist, 161
Pharmacokineticist, 71
Pharmacologist, 26
Pharmocology, 88
PharmaTrack™, 239
Phase I-III, 5, 88
Physician panel, 19, 28
Physician (see Investigator)
Placebo, 57
Plan-Do-Check approach, 13
Planned closure, 46

Planning checklist, 35, 50
Planning, importance of, 2, 113
PocketTrials software, 239
Postmarketing, 228, 232
Power of a test, 67, 231
Power and Precision software, 244
Precision, 64, 192, 211
Pre-design checklist, 35
Predictors, finding, 217
Pretrial meetings, 168
Preventive measures, 43, 79
Procedure manuals, 24, 83, 95ff, 163, 179
Profit considerations, 72
Program documentation, 99, 218
Program testing, 27, 136
Programmers
  screen preparation, 26, 127
  statistical, 30
Programming conventions, 136
Project management software, 180, 238
Project manager, 23, 168, 180, 230
Proposals,
  objectives, 89
  reviewing and rewriting, 49
  clinical overview, 86
Protocol
  deviations, 42, 78, 171, 178, 204
  table of contents, 87
Pull-down menus, 129
p-value, 223

Quality control, 42, 47, 91, 123, 179
Quality-of-life, 49

Radio button, 128
Randomization, 56
  blocked, 59
  response adaptive, 72
  stratified, 60
Randomized trials, 58

Rank tests, 223
Reactions, severe, 171
Recruiting
  factors in, 113
  media campaigns, 1114
  monitoring, 77
  patients, 112
  problems with, 29
  physicians, 108
  targeting, 70
  tracking, 176–177
Redundant variables,
Regulatory agencies
  advice, 11
  approval of, 19, 25, 163
  notification, 79
  requirements, 57
  submissions to, 9, 83, 102
Regulatory liaison, 25
Relational database, 146,
Repeated tests, 214
Reports
  clinical overview, 86
  start with, 7, 45
  topics covered by, 97–102, 189
  "Rescue efforts," costs of, 188
Resource center guide, 110
Response adaptive randomization, 72
Review committees, 29, 30, 163, 179, 183–185
Run-in period, 117–118

SaberTooth Curriculum, 213
Safety
  measures, 18
  monitoring board, 48
  trials, 5
Sample determination
  formulas for, 64
Samples
  requirements, 216
  representative,
  size, 8, 36, 63
  cost, 72
SAS
  analysis, 196, 200, 202

software, 238, 243
  univariate procedure, 181
Screen-capture utilities, 137
Screen development, 124–131
Security, 155–158
Sequential tests, 185
Servers, 150
Sham surgery, 58
Side effects
  anticipated, 39
Significance level, 66, 223
Silicon implants, 4, 58
Silktest software, 137, 245
Simpson's paradox, 210
Site (see Treatment site)
Smirnov test, 208
Smoking, 127
Software
  checklist, 162
  developer, 26
  documentation, 218
Speech recognition, 239
Sponsor data, 88
Spreadsheets, 144
SPSS, 243
SQL, 147
SQL-Amywhere®, 151
Staff turnover, 171
Staffing, 23
Standard error, 192
Stata©, 181, 243
Statistical
  analysis, 91, 103, 194
  assumptions, 216
  programmers, 30
  significance, 209, 217
  software, 243
  terminology, 222
Statistics checklist, 213
StatXact software, 243
Stenosis, 39
Stratified randomization, 59
Stress testing, 138
Student's t, 223
Study (see, also, Clinical trials)
  committees, 93
  closure, 46

justification, 88
  objectives, 37
  population, 44, 203
  protocol, table of contents, 87
  time lines, 45
StudyBuilder software, 240
Subgroup hypotheses, 5, 232
Subjects, (see Patients)
Subsamples, 69
Supplies, 161, 176
Support
  technical, 140
Surrogate response, 38–39
Survival data, 200
Sybase InfoMaker, 240
Sybase SQL Anywhere, 242
SyMetric software, 243
S+SeqTrial, 244

Teaching hospitals, 109
Team roles, 32
Technical design decisions,
Technical support, 140
Technical writers, 26
Tertiary end points, 41
Testing
  database, 158
  equivalence, 209
  software, 20, 136–138
Testing leads, 27
Test phase checklist, 163–164
Third-party facilitator, 229
Time line, 45
Time-to-event data, 65, 200
Touch screen software, 239
Toxicity, investigating, 186
Training program, 20, 43, 78, 139
Transnational trials, 3, 30, 36–7
Treatment
  allocation, 47, 50, 60
  code cracking, 47, 62, 77
  discontinuing, (see Closure)

modifications, 79, 185
noncompliance with, 170
plan or regimen, 90
TrialXS software, 237
Treatment sites
  coordinators, 28, 75, 163, 206
  number, 36, 70
  selecting, 107
  visits, 111, 139, 165, 69
Trial review committee, 230
Trials (see, Clinical Trials)
TrialWorks™ software, 238

Triple blinding, 62
t-test procedure, 195, 200, 223
Type I and II errors, 66, 223
Type-and-verify field, 129

Validate, 1, 103, 129
Variability measures, 103
Variable and fixed costs, 229
Variation
  coping with, 55
  minimizing, 96
  individual-to-individual

VIP patient treatment, 116
Volunteers, attracting, 113

Web-based data entry, 154–155
Westfall procedure, 215
Wilcoxon test, 198, 223
Winrunner software, 137, 245
Withdrawals (see Dropouts)

Zelen's test, 196, 204